God's House Calls

Finding God Through My Patients

Jim Roach, M.D.

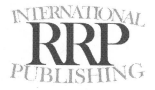

RRP International Publishing LLC
Richmond/Lexington, Ky.

RRP International LLC, DBA Eugenia Ruth LLC
330 Eastern Bypass
Ste #1 Box 302
Richmond, Ky. 40475

www.rrpinternational.org

DISCLAIMER

Neither the author nor the publisher is engaged in rendering professional advice or services to the individual reader. This book is not intended as a substitute for the medical advice of integrative health practitioners. The reader should regularly consult an integrative health practitioner in matters relating to his/her health and particularly with respect to any symptoms that may require diagnosis or medical attention. Neither the author nor the publisher shall be liable or responsible for any loss, injury or damage allegedly arising from any information or suggestion contained in this book.

All of the events contained in this book were told to Dr. Roach personally through the course of his medical practice, communications or travels. All efforts have been made to ensure the accuracy of the information contained in this book as of the date of publication. Some names and identifying information have been changed to protect the privacy of the individuals discussed in this book while leaving intact the essential details of each narrative. But know that events like these happen on a regular basis to people of all backgrounds from all parts of the world. They are just rarely discussed publicly and openly...until now.

ISBN-13: 978-0-9793644-4-0

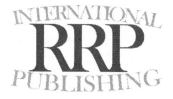

Previous Books:

Take More Naps (And 100 Other Life Lessons)

The Art of Opinion Writing: Insider Secrets from Top Op-Ed Columnists

The Art of Column Writing: Insider Secrets from Art Buchwald, Dave Barry, Arianna Huffington, Pete Hamill and Other Great Columnists

Don McNay's Greatest Hits: Ten Years as an Award-Winning Columnist

Life Lessons from Cancer

Son of a Son of a Gambler: Joe McNay 80th Birthday Edition

Life Lessons from the Golf Course: The Quest for Spiritual Meaning, Psychological Understanding and Inner Peace through the Game of Golf

Life Lessons from the Lottery: Protecting Your Money in a Scary World

Wealth Without Wall Street: A Main Street Guide to Making Money

www.rrpinternational.org

Dedication

This is dedicated to my wife who God provided - a devoted, loving partner who has given me two incredible children.

Table of Contents

Foreword

"It must've been wild angels, wild angels
Watching over you and me.
Wild angels, wild angels
Baby, what else could it be?"
-Martina McBride

It could have been a wild angel that connected me to Dr. Jim Roach, M.D., but that angel came in the form of an 88-year-old journalist named Al Smith.

Al is one of the greatest living Kentuckians and my journalism mentor, but I thought in November 2009 that he was hitting the finish line. My garage had two small steps and when he came to visit, we had to carry him up them. He looked bad. Al spends his winters in Sarasota, Florida. When he came back in April 2010, he was in high spirits and invited me to lunch at the Bangkok House, which is at the bottom of a steep flight of steps near the University of Kentucky campus. It wasn't until we started to leave that I noticed that Al was basically skipping up the long flight of steps.

When I asked him what caused the turnaround, he credited Dr. Jim and the regime of supplements, vitamins and diet changes that Dr. Jim recommended.

Al turned 88 in January. He is still writing, speaking out and maintaining a busy travel schedule. After I saw what Jim did for Al, I became one of Jim's patients and his friend.

Dr. Jim is one of the nation's leaders in a concept called Integrative Medicine. Jim combines his medical school education and decades of daily practice as a family doctor with an approach that combines a variety of concepts. It is all designed to help a person live a longer and healthier life. Dr. Roach and his team at the Midway Center for Integrative Medicine will often spend a couple of hours with a patient. Seeing how many medical corporations are forcing their doctors to practice like they are on a time clock, Dr. Jim is a refreshing change from the medical experience that many people endure. He is as far away from the "seven minutes and prescribe the latest pills" style as you can get.

Dr. Jim and his team get to know their patients on a deep and personal level. Located in genteel horse country, The Midway Center is a glimpse of what the practice of medicine was like in the days of small town doctors and house calls, but Midway has all the latest research and cutting edge technology at their fingertips. Dr. Jim is all over the United States, doing lectures, going to high powered conferences and interacting with the biggest experts in the Integrative Medicine field.

I contacted him when I was in a desperate mode to find a way to have weight loss surgery. I weighed 377 pounds and knew that I had to make a dramatic move. Dr. Roach is not one to push patients into surgery, but recognized I was a unique case. I'll tell more of my story in a series of books called *Project 199: My Business Plan to Lose 175 Pounds*, but Jim was instrumental in getting me to the right surgeon, Dr. Derek Weiss, for a successful operation. I just turned 56 and I'm in the best health of my adult life.

When he was helping me, Dr. Jim mentioned he was writing a book. As a publisher, I assumed Jim was writing a book about his work in Integrative Medicine and immediately became interested. Anything he wrote about his medical practice would be a big hit.

Thus, I was taken aback when he said that his book was spiritual in nature.

I might have been more taken aback if I had not had my own story:

"If only you believe like I believe, we'd get by
If only you believe in miracles, so would I"
-Jefferson Starship

On Saturday February 27, 1993, my father was terminally ill with prostate cancer in Cincinnati and I was in my apartment in Lexington, Kentucky, getting ready to go to a University of Kentucky basketball game.

About nine a.m., my telephone started making a strange kind of ring. My answering machine picked up on four rings, but it rang several times more before I could get to it and pick it up. I heard a voice on the other end which sounded a little like my father at the other end of a tunnel yelling, "Don! Don! I need you, I need you."

Then there was a click.

I frantically started calling his home and the phone kept ringing and ringing. After about 20 minutes or so, my frazzled stepmother picked up the phone, told me that my dad's heart had stopped earlier and they were waiting for the ambulance.

Dad couldn't have called me. He probably was not actually alive. They paddled him back to life and brought him to the emergency room at Christ Hospital in Cincinnati.

The "call" gave me a chance to ditch the basketball game and drive as fast as I could to the hospital in Cincinnati. When I got there, a number of family members and friends were there and a moment later, they wheeled Dad in on a gurney. He gave me a thumbs up, like former Reagan Press Secretary Jim Brady did after he was shot, and they took him back into another room. He died a few minutes later as they got my stepmother and I to agree to end artificial measures to keep him alive. No funeral mass site had been selected or a funeral home. I made all those arrangements while his body sat there cold, in the same room with me.

When Dad became sick, I started praying constantly and he started praying as well. I went back to church for the first time in a decade. As death approached, he really wanted to connect back to the Catholic Church that he had left decades earlier. A bishop who was a friend of mine and then a local priest walked through the complicated process of rejoining the church and receiving sacraments. He did it. A few weeks before he died, the local priest walked Dad through confession, last rites, communion and all the other things so that Dad could have a funeral mass and be buried in the Catholic Church.

My father had been a bookie and well-known professional gambler. As Billy Joel would say, he ran with "a dangerous crowd, they ain't too pretty, they ain't too proud." He also befriended some of the most important leaders and sports stars in Cincinnati. His funeral mass had about 400 people attend and it was painfully obvious that 390 had never been in a church before. The crowd ranged from Mafia chiefs to police chiefs, but they sent Dad on his trip to heaven, even if some were going to need a lot of prayers and repentance if they were ever going to get there themselves.

I spent years trying to find a logical explanation for the "call" from Dad. We carefully checked the phone records, but there was no record and there was no physical way he could have made that call at that moment. It also did not record on my answering machine.

Without the "call," I would have gone to the basketball game and in those days before mobile devices, it would have been many hours after the death before I found out. I wouldn't have seen him that last time, I would not have been there for the decision on the life support, and I would not have been there to arrange for the funeral and funeral mass.

Dad needed me and it was obvious that he used a voice from beyond, rather than AT&T, to get in touch.

It was not the first time, or last, I got a call from beyond.

I had a previous experience in high school where my mother won a $1000 drawing with the winning number of 1313 (I was born on Friday the 13th), and I knew and told her the night *before* she was going to win. I had dreamt the previous night that our track coach would call the house. When he actually called, I was waiting for him. He called to tell us Mom had won. I was on his team for four years and never got another call.

In 1994, I rolled over in bed and told my wife, "Theresa had her baby." A couple of hours later, my mother called and told us about the birth. It was at the exact second that I rolled over in bed and announced it.

I take it seriously when someone tells the type of stories that Dr. Jim discusses in this book. Something supernatural happened to me. More than once. I'm not a weekly churchgoer or a religious leader. What happened was very real and there is no explanation, short of a spiritual one, as to what happened in my life.

Dr. Jim is doing us a great service; he is getting these incidents into the public forum in an unvarnished and unabashed way.

I understand why patients told Dr. Jim and probably never told anyone else. Jim is a man of ramrod integrity, but also very easy to connect with (he is Dr. Jim, not Dr. Roach). He earns the respect that comes from his lifetime of medical practice and community service. You can't help but trust him. His patients have the rare opportunity to have a conversation with a family doctor that lasts longer than a minute. He is a question asker and a researcher, not someone dictating orders. People trust him with their deepest secrets. He has a quiet confidence that allows you to want to open up and talk. I've written several books (two are bestsellers specifically about my father) and written hundreds of newspaper columns, but never wrote about the "call" from my dad. I'm normally one who will speak out, but this is a topic that seemed a little sensitive.

Dr. Roach gave me the courage to "put it out in the street." Just as many others are now telling their story to a public audience.

As Dr. Jim has often quoted, "When people talk to God, they call it prayer. When God talks to you, they call it schizophrenia."

Now I know that if I am crazy, there are a lot of other crazy people with me.

Dr. Jim has done a great service by getting us to put our experiences out in the open. And finding out that hundreds (probably thousands) of others have their own unique story to tell.

God's House Calls will be the beginning of a snowball of people having the courage to share experiences like those in the book. We learn a lot from Jim's patients, but we really learn a lot from Dr. Jim.

"Well, I won't back down
No, I won't back down .
You can stand me up at the gates of hell
But I won't back down"
-Tom Petty (and a later hit by Johnny Cash.)

It would have been easy for Dr. Jim to have skipped this book or written another book instead. He is a well-respected physician. He's built a tremendous medical practice and has the sense of grace and manners of someone who grew up in horse country with a family that owned a famous and successful horse farm. His late father Ben and his late brother Tom, along with famed horse breeder William Farrish, bred the 1999 Kentucky Derby winner Charismatic at their well-known Parrish Hill Farm. Charismatic won the Preakness and ran third after breaking his leg at his Triple Crown attempt at the Belmont. The farm also bred Princess Rooney, a winner at the Kentucky Oaks and in the inaugural Breeders Cup.

Jim has a strong devotion to his wife and two children. He and Dee Dee were married on July 3, 1976 and work together every day at the Midway Center. To see them, you would think they are still on their honeymoon, and they have a love and devotion to be admired. Both of his children are excellent people and have successful careers. His son James is a meritorious attorney in Ohio and his daughter Liz has been a speechwriter and assistant to Kentucky Governor Steve Beshear.

Jim learned about more than horses from his family. He learned the art of giving back. His father, Dr. Ben Roach, was the founder of the Markey Cancer Center at the University of the Kentucky, one of the top cancer centers in the region. Jim also learned from his family to do good deeds quietly. Although there is a building as part of the Markey Center named for Dr. Ben Roach, the center is not. Jim's mother, a civic activist extraordinaire, was killed in a car crash on New Year's Eve several years ago, as she was delivering baskets of food to poor people and drove off an icy and snowy road. Jim was one of the first advocates of a statewide smoking ban in Kentucky and an early leader in Habitat for Humanity in Kentucky.

One of Dr. Jim's great heroes was Millard Fuller, the founder of Habitat for Humanity. He took a simple idea and a focused message and built an organization that made a huge impact on the world.

I could see Jim doing something as big as Habitat. He has the same type of drive, commitment and passion that Mr. Fuller had. Also, he has the ability to focus the organization on the mission and not on the leader.

As a person, I deeply admire Dr. Jim. As a publisher, I was quite concerned. His low-key, self-effacing, "don't brag on yourself" philosophy that is so ingrained in who he is also makes it hard to sell books. I've written several best-selling books, but I am always aware that people like Paris Hilton and reality show stars have sold far more books than I have. Taking off your clothes or doing something outlandish seems to be the best way to draw attention to a book.

My odds of getting Dr. Roach to take his clothes off in public were very slim. I wasn't going to go there.

Then it hit me that Dr. Jim has two things going for him. One is that he views this book as an act of evangelism, rather than an opportunity to talk about himself. Jim sees the book as a calling and a cause, and books are the way to get his message out.

Secondly, Dr. Jim is a rebel. A quiet, self-effacing rebel who grew up on a horse farm and studied at Duke University, like his father and brother did, but a rebel nonetheless.

It would have been easy for Dr. Jim to keep rolling along, handing out pills and practicing the same kind of medicine that most family care doctors do. See a lot of patients, hand out a lot of prescription drugs. Instead, Dr. Jim created an entirely new medical model. He promotes healthy living, vitamins and supplements over prescription medicines. He focuses on breaking edge information and seems to be doing research and studies on the latest trends 24 hours a day. Not many doctors schedule two and a half hour visits with their patients or test for allergies and ailments that no one ever heard of or thought about. Jim does.

Dr. Jim, spawned from the most conventional of backgrounds, is an unconventional man. He took a lot of cheap shots from the traditional medical community when he changed his practice to one that works exceptionally well. He took on unpopular causes, like trying to implement a statewide smoking ban in a tobacco state like Kentucky, long before anyone dreamed that would be possible.

Thus, speaking out and writing this book doesn't surprise me. He has put together an exceptional book based around firm belief and vision. He will go all-out to get people interested in what he has to say. Negative reviews won't bother him and may push him to work harder. He has a mission and he is going to fulfill it.

As the song says, "he won't back down."

I'm honored and proud to be part of this.

Don McNay, CLU, ChFC, MSFS, CSSC,
Best-selling author, former nationally syndicated business columnist,
Huffington Post contributor
www.mcnayconsulting.com

Introduction

When writing this book, there was a temptation to whitewash its contents, to conform to a particular spiritual belief system. That would have made it tidy and more acceptable to a traditional audience.

But I do not sense that as my calling. What for me is most amazing, and continually emphasized by these stories, is God is bigger than we can ever understand. The complexities of God are largely beyond our knowing.

So while we, for our rational purposes, like to put God into a box that completely conforms to our own logic and interpretations, what I am learning is that God cannot be confined by our desires or our limitations.

Perhaps my biggest revelation was stated simply by a patient. God is very creative. God does not communicate in simple mundane ways. God communicates in exceedingly creative ways. The "stamp of approval" that is indeed God is the overwhelming, loving presence we feel when God communicates. It is also the appropriateness of the message, which hits home when we see the manifestation of God's love in action.

Most may believe that the Bible is complete in its message. But our Bible differs from the original. In the centuries after the Bible's first organization, some books were removed. Was this divine or political? It is alleged that Constantine in 350AD promised a throat slashing and confiscation of all property for Christians believing in reincarnation; supportive books of the Bible were removed. In just a little beyond my lifetime, the Apocrypha, always an addition to the Bible, has been removed due to influential individuals "tidying it up."

I am not a theological scholar, do not pretend to be all knowing and do not trust anyone who says they have all the answers. God is too big. God is too creative.

As these stories are presented, their inclusion is not because I know for certain they are real or are always consistent with my reality. They are included because my patients and friends found them to have personal spiritual significance. Their lives were substantially impacted by these events, always in a positive way.

Perhaps in judging what is right and wrong, what is truth and not truth, we need to consider Jesus' comment that we will know it by the fruit that it bears. Do these events bear good fruit in the lives of those so touched?

Perhaps the mark of truth is that all of my patients have felt blessed by these events. They are now more spiritual. They are more intuitive. They are more connected to God. Their beliefs have been girded. It is witnessed to me by their spiritual presence. It is witnessed to me by their love.

Understanding Possibility

Albert Einstein learned that a particle separated into two components moving in opposite directions, despite the distance apart, have a direct, immediate influence on each other. Even when they are on opposite sides of the universe, what influences one precisely influences the other. They are connected somewhat as if by a cord. They have eternal, instant relationship. He called that "spooky behavior." Particles in each of us have an infinite relationship with the universe. Are we forever connected to its central force, God?

Einstein's introduction of quantum theory was expanded to recognize that particles are constantly alternating with waveforms. Viewing them influences this process. We are not persistent solid mass, but rather a fluctuating energy form.

A great distance, relative to their size, separates these alternating subatomic forms. Understanding this helps us recognize that we are in essence 99 percent space, or perhaps 99.99 percent space. Thus the amount of solid mass in our body is less than our fist. We are largely hot air. It is not the mass that gives us "solidity," but the strength of the energy fields they create.

In fact, everything we encounter is also an energy field. Our visual and tactile senses lie to us.

Picture our bodies as a more solid version of clouds. Clouds separate into two. Later, the two may reunite. This aids visualizing a spiritual energy field separating from a "physical" one and reconnecting.

During medical training, my left brain was crammed full of facts. My right brain, the intuitive side, was neglected. In essence, we were taught to only believe what our five senses could detect, only what our tests demonstrate. Anything not fitting into that paradigm was psychosomatic or neurotic. Many patients fit into that category. Since our professors taught state-of-the-art medicine, if we as doctors did not know it, it likely did not exist and patients were consciously or subconsciously fabricating it. Everything was atoms, molecules and DNA.

While our brain energy field is small, extending not much beyond our skull, our heart energy field extends out fifteen feet. A heart tracing EKG measurement can be achieved at that distance.

The heart, which I was taught was muscle, is in fact half nerve tissue. The heart has a memory and interacts regularly with the brain. It is now well documented that heart transplants change the personality of the recipient toward one similar to the giver. We are learning that who we are is more heart than brain.

When approaching 50, I wanted to see how long and well I could live. I have now attended dozens of conferences not associated with pharmaceutical interventions. The first 20 years of my practice I put patients on more and more medicine. The last 14 years I have been pulling them off medicine as fast as I can with far greater success, utilizing comprehensive assessment including genetics, micronutrients, heavy metals, hormones and food sensitivities while focusing on optimal nutrition, safe interventions including botanicals and now spiritual perspective.

These groundbreaking conferences taught understanding and utilization of quantum physics, which has yet to significantly impact the medical field. As energy fields, we become open to a large number of phenomena that previously seemed incomprehensible. Our spiritual energy field enters our body before birth and exits after death. What you will learn as you read these stories is that the soul is sometimes restless or frankly scared, and may choose to leave the body at times during our life and then reconnect. It is most common in childhood, during childbirth, trauma, surgery and near-death, but can occur even when overjoyed or spontaneously.

A few years ago this concept to me bordered on the incredulous. But as I hear reports from patients on an almost daily basis, I recognize their validity.

In sharing this with a retired doctor, he exclaimed he had never heard this from his patients in all of the years of his practice. The reason, however, is simple. He did not ask. And he did not have the level of trust needed.

Someone sharing out-of-body experiences must have confidence their report will not be ridiculed and that they will not be placed in a mental institution. As these stories come from my serene, upbeat patients who I would want as best friends or next-door neighbors, I respect their authenticity. Learning that we are hot air helps in that understanding.

So as you read these stories, you are welcome to keep one foot in the conventional world. But place the other foot firmly in the world that Einstein has opened for us.

Since the entire universe is energy, that catapults the possibilities. We are malleable. We can transform and be transformed. Healing can occur rapidly.

All of life has vibrancy. Ice is of low vibration, steam of high vibration. The higher our vibration, the more we can transform.

The vibrancy we emit impacts our environment. Sending high vibrations to water results in positive, high energy molecular formations. Sending low vibrations leads to chaotic molecular arrangement.

Love has a high vibration character, and hate is low vibration. The energy we bring to others either brightens or dampens their energy field or "spirit." We are spiritual beings.

This information may strike you as bizarre. For others it may seem "unscientific." But I invite you to just be open to the possibility both in your mind and in your heart. Leave that door open as you hear these stories.

After finishing this book, validate this for yourself. If you can approach others with an open heart and gain their confidence, whole new worlds will open up to you. For these are not the experiences of the few. These are the experiences of the many.

These events are transformative. Those in darkness now bask in light. Suddenly, whatever happens to them in this earthly realm is of lesser importance. They have not just faith, but a "knowing" that they are a part of something much bigger. They know that their life is now about a mission. They have meaning. What we do matters. It is all about one word: Love.

My Story – I Could Never Have Imagined

My patients have directed my spiritual pathway, leading to mystical experience and a tremendous appreciation of God's love and creativity.

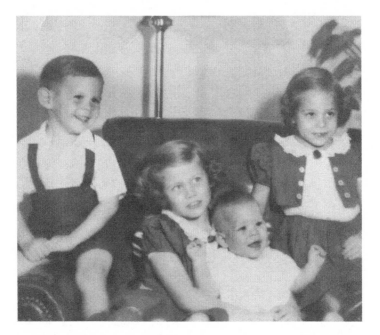

Growing up in a small town in central Kentucky, thoroughbred horses would race through the fields. The smell of tobacco wafted from the barns. Riding your bike through town, people might call you by your last name: "Hey Roach!" I felt the love.

My grandfather "Bapa" was the spiritual leader of the family. While doing postgraduate work at Harvard, he was watching a play when it was suddenly interrupted. His name was called due to an emergency at sea. Bapa was needed to open the special laboratory to receive

Morse code messages from a tragic event. The Titanic had sunk. The transmission listed passengers who had died.

Named as the first state Bridge Engineer for Georgia, he insisted on the highest quality work. Governor Eugene Tallmadge had other ideas, insisting unscrupulous patronage friends do the work. Bapa, firm in his religious and ethical beliefs, was fired for non-compliance. They had to lift him in his chair, carting him from the building. This led to a highly successful career as an independent contractor, overseeing bridge construction all over Georgia.

When visiting Decatur, Georgia on vacations, my family would kneel at bedtime for family prayers. Bapa would pray for our leaders that they might have wisdom in their decisions. He would pray for family unity. Bapa would always finish with the Lord's Prayer.

On Sunday mornings, we grandchildren had to recite a memorized verse of Scripture before eating our melon and plowing into our waffles. My older brother Tom used "Jesus wept," but that only worked once.

In a pivotal moment, Bapa's close friend, Mr. Friedman, had a near-death experience following a car accident where he was thrown from his vehicle into a ditch. Fortunately, his secretary was in the car behind him. She rushed to her boss, who was unconscious. She slapped him and yelled, "Wake Up!" His indignant response: "I don't want to wake up!"

Mr. Friedman told my Grandfather, "Searcy, don't ever worry about dying. Dying is the easiest thing you will ever do."

"Dying is the easiest thing you will ever do."

* * * * *

College summers were spent at Woodford Hospital. After starting my medical practice, it became my second home for the next 20 years.

During a hospital crisis in 2001, its survival fell into my hands. A board member "assured" me, "Jim, there is nothing to be done." I was indignant. "That may be your reality, but it is not mine!"

Two days before the hospital was to permanently close on a Monday morning, I rounded at Taylor Manor. My heart poured into prayer. Before a TV camera, I pled for hospital survival. God was listening.

In the middle of that night, I woke suddenly with a plan. All we needed was money! And I lived in the richest county in the state. The next day, in a truly miraculous fashion, it came together. I asked a friend to gather a group of horsemen to arrange the essential financial support. Then strategists were called to a "Sunday School" meeting at one of their homes. The camaraderie and positive energy of the strategists led promptly to a plan that would not even require financial support – extremely fortunate since the horsemen financier meeting fell through. For the hospital, it was a new beginning.

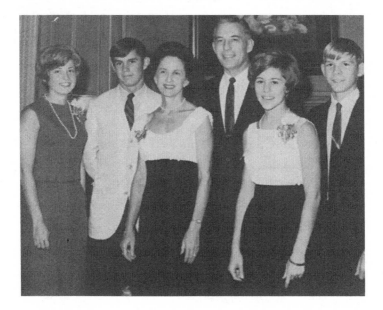

* * * * *

In 2006, my wife Dee Dee and I joined an integrative holistic medicine conference at the peaceful Crossings near Austin. At their bookstore, I was entranced by melodic gong music. On a walk, we heard the identical musical gongs in the wind. Synchronicity. We were exactly where we were supposed to be on life's pathway.

* * * * *

At their next ABIHM event in Virginia, I rose to ask about my shoulder injury. Afterwards, an oriental Reiki master asked if I desired healing. "Of course!"

We retreated to a quiet spot. With his hands above my shoulders, he asked me to vocalize whatever came to mind. From somewhere, words appeared. "My mother died suddenly in a car accident New Year's Eve. I never got to say goodbye." Tears formed in my eyes.

Afterwards, my shoulder felt the same. But the next morning, it was completely well.

My shoulder healed overnight through Reiki

* * * * *

The National Publicity Summit in New York City was an opportunity to meet the media. While there, I met Dru from Calgary. She was excited that I was from Kentucky. Al, an executive there, had been wrongly accused of corporate crime. He was dying of cancer. "You must tell him it is not his time to die!"

Yes, I was supposed to visit a multimillionaire stranger dying from cancer to enlighten him that it was not his time. Was she crazy?

"You must tell him it is not his time to die!"

Back home, I called a friend who knew Al. Weeks earlier, Al had been admitted to hospice. "Too late," I thought. But then hospice released him.

My friend joining me, there I was at Al's house. Al lay in bed in a semi-comatose state. At least it was not Lazarus. As I shared Dru's message, Al stirred. Then he sat up. He walked to the window. Now he was conversing with his family and friend!

Al stayed active for weeks, but he and the family chose not to utilize most of my anti-cancer remedies. Al died one month after my visit.

* * * * *

One night I had a dream of a large hovering wave getting ready to crash on me. It was frozen in place while business went on as usual below. Certainly I could make a case for impending doom from the dream. The dream was so unusual and real, I shared it with my wife that morning.

At work, my wife discovered we had a major financial issue that caught us totally off guard. I was two hours behind seeing patients most of the day. The last patient yelled at me without provocation and walked out. That may have happened to a lesser degree once 20 years earlier.

I did not finish office notes and leave the office until 9:23 p.m. On our shortened walk, very unusually my wife had only critical things to say. She went to bed without saying goodnight. The dream had proven prophetic for how the day was to go.

But as always, when we notice, good things happen, too. A new nurse practitioner, in for her first day of work, had a perfect demeanor. One of my patients with chronic fatigue, fibromyalgia AND a fever could not have been nicer; she did not demonstrate an inkling of the issues affecting her and seemed an angel personified. So that night, throughout the walk, I sent "thank you's" to Jesus. Ever since that challenging day, life has been much better.

* * * * *

In a dream, I was sitting in my usual spot at church, the second row of pews on the left where we have sat for two decades. A bright light appeared from the upper right. A soap-like bubble emerged. It got progressively larger. Finally, detail emerged.

Inside the bubble was the softly smiling face of my Grandmother Roach. She looked about 60 years old as I remembered her. The bubble got close to my face, nearly filling my field of vision. It was radiating heat. I could feel her physical warmth. The impression was very strong. Never had I had a dream emanating heat.

Physical heat was the seal that this dream was sending a message

For a few moments, her bubble lingered. I soaked it in. It was very real. Gently the bubble then floated upward. Transforming into a moth, it then flew toward the ceiling and faded away.

Grandmother Roach had suffered from bipolar disorder, requiring treatment with electroconvulsive therapy. Recently, I had been utilizing progressive approaches in treating a patient with manic-depression. This was a message, a "thank you" acknowledging an important purpose of my earthly journey. The exuding warmth was the seal that it was real.

* * * * *

Between the ages of six and 13, Marcia had three near-death experiences. She became very intuitive, perhaps as a result of those experiences. Marcia can connect in directly for messages through a dream-state that she can self-induce. Notice I did not say, "She reports that she can."

She lived in Colorado with her husband. A persistent message would come to Marcia. It was the word "Ashland," always associated with the picture of a college on a hill. The message haunted her. It would not let loose. As a powerful message, she felt obligated to find the answer.

Marcia visited Ashland, Oregon seeking an explanation. Lithia Park, the highest water source of calming natural lithium, was lovely. But teenagers there were lost souls, she lamented.

My spiritual guide appears

Marcia then moved to Frankfort, Kentucky and saw me as a new patient. When she searched YouTube for "Dr. Roach" and "Ashland," she made an interesting discovery. In a video, I was giving a testimonial for the Mederi Foundation. It was while I had been visiting Ashland, Oregon.

In Midway, she discovered Midway College. It sat on a hill and corresponded to the vision in her message. Her conclusion: I was the connection.

Marcia did not have an appointment, but insisted on being seen. Normally we cannot help in those situations, but my receptionist wife sensed something different about this request.

When I walked into the patient room, Marcia looked up

apprehensively. "You are probably going to think that I am crazy, but there is something that I just have to tell you." Her story poured out.

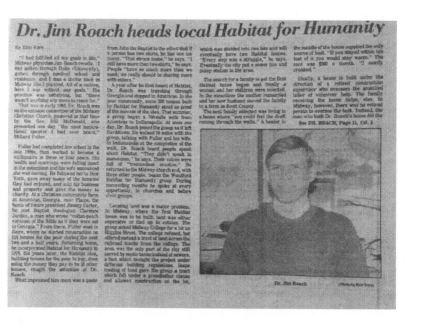

Dr. Jim Roach heads local Habitat for Humanity

From my Quantum Leap coaching, I recognized that a life mission was to educate health practitioners. Through 10,000 hours of study over 14 years, my integrative health knowledge had blossomed. As a consequence, I planned my first educational event. A website had been developed, but the event location had not been announced. I had decided, in my mind, it would be at Midway College.

But I was getting concerned. The conference had a big price tag. What if no one came? In fact, only two had signed up.

Marcia first asked to see my hands. On my right hand, she gently examined the second finger, then the third. Finally the fourth, then back to the third. What she discerned appeared to reaffirm the message she was about to share. I could sense her spiritual essence.

Marcia told me that I was having an event the middle of next month.

It was going to be at Midway College. "What you are doing is supposed to happen." I was doing the right thing by going forward with this event.

"Whoever is behind this message is very powerful"

Marcia said the message was strong. Whoever was behind it was very powerful. It had led her to visit Ashland, Oregon. It caused her and her husband to move from Colorado to Frankfort, KY. Then "coincidentally" she met me. She saw Midway College on the edge of my town. It was all for the purpose of delivering this message.

She urged me to meditate daily at the same time, using my thumb and index or fifth finger. These are the ones tuned into auditory. Say "Ohm" and listen for messages. My messages will come through the auditory. I am not to focus on visual or kinesthetic cues as much.

Marcia sensed that I am a very intuitive person. She could see an aura around me. Marcia also saw it temporarily change when I at first looked puzzled.

At one point Marcia was afraid to tell me all of this. What would I, a physician she barely knew, think about her message? How would I, a well-educated man, take this unusual set of occurrences?

I reassured her. Yes, I was ready for this message. On receiving it, I teared up. It was a question I had been asking for weeks. It was an endpoint from my travels to New York and Philadelphia. It was incredibly reaffirming.

More practitioners signed up for my event. A total of six attended. There was an impressively positive energy. We shared a special dinner at Holly Hill Inn. Stories were traded. We all sensed the importance of our gathering.

Six months later I repeated the event. Seventeen attended, from

California to New Jersey, Texas to Wisconsin with 10 states represented. It was also very special. One attendee, Sue Massie, N.D., was one of the most spiritually gifted I have ever met.

* * * * *

My spiritual leader reappeared in early June. She said that I needed to locate a "ledger-like" report in which is denoted a project started by an uncle. I am to find it and finish what he started. There are students in the Midway area that are being mislabeled as incapable or underachievers; my goal is to identify and help them.

I am to be a leader. Currently I am operating in a circular motion "like a figure of eight." It is time to break out, to do the mission I am supposed to do.

It was "written in stone" that I was to write a book on spiritual stories

When I told Marcia I was considering writing a book on spiritual stories, "it is already written in stone" that I will be writing that book she shared. Six weeks later, when mentioning spiritual stories to a friend, he surprised me by saying he wanted to publish them.

* * * * *

When my prostate PSA level soared years ago, I panicked. Mentored by Donnie Yance, America's best botanical medicine expert with 30 years of cancer experience, and Dwight McKee, M.D., the top integrative oncologist in the country, I have at least double outcomes in nearly all cancer patients who followed full protocols. But me?

Putting my tools to work, closely monitoring my PSA, I chipped away until it had dropped 80 percent. God put me in the shoes of a prostate cancer patient to learn important ways to manage it.

Then one breast enlarged near a sensitized nipple. While breast cancer in men is uncommon, how could I know for sure? Donnie, at a sidewalk café in Scottsdale, offered complete reassurance: it was the estrogen influence of my smoothie's pea protein powder. Genes, foods and some supplements contributed to the net estrogen impact. God knew this was important for me in managing estrogen cancers.

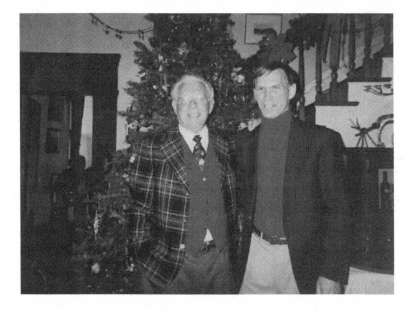

Lyme disease is highly prevalent. While conventional testing is insensitive, the proper assessment revealed half of my chronic fatigue and fibromyalgia patients might have Lyme, as did most of my Parkinson's, multiple sclerosis, Tourette's and benign essential tremor patients. Difficulty focusing the eyes that fluctuates, light or noise sensitivity are common distinguishing features.

My son on an overnight camping trip used a protective spray. I did not and landed 100 insect bites (my son, zero). I developed a mild right hand tremor with poor handwriting. Learning strategies to improve this once again benefited the Lyme patients I manage.

In Ecuador after missing supper, I arrived with my son at our motel at cliff edge a mile above the small city below. Instinctively washing off fruit left for us in the room, I indulged. That resulted in a severe parasitic gastroenteritis. But as long as I didn't eat or drink, I felt fine. Strangely I realized that in time, I would pleasantly fade away.

Could death be pleasant?

When swallowing supplements, I didn't see the plastic cylindrical preservative. For minutes I choked uncontrollably. It hit me that I should be panicking. Instead, a peaceful feeling settled in. Lowering my head to the ground, gravity removed the intruder. Could death be a pleasant destination? The lesson I later learned: it depends.

* * * * *

After one of my Sunday school classes on near-death experiences, Kenna approached me. During the class she had felt the presence of my mother. Mom had died 20 years earlier and never met Kenna.

"Your Mom wants you to know she appreciates what you are doing with the class. She is pleased with your work at church and spirituality." Kenna continued, "Your mother is a very warm, gentle, open soul. She is not a big woman." With her mouth twisted and left eye squinted, Kenna also noted, "She has a Southern accent." Nailed her!

Kenna channels my mother

* * * * *

Eva Walters hugged my mother, Ruth, at Thanksgiving. As she did so, she heard a voice in her head. Eva recognized the voice. It was God's. The voice told her Ruth would die in six weeks.

Six weeks later, my mother's car veered off a country road into a fence. She had been delivering food to needy families. It was New Year's Eve. Hours later, she died

It was during her first visit to my office that Eva told me this story. It was New Year's Eve, exactly 19 years after my Mom's death.

––––––

Late in the following spring, my mother came to Eva in a dream. Ruth was in her vintage car full of gifts. "Eva, you need to convey a message to my son Tom. Tell him to do what was in his heart."

Eva, knowing that this was a divine message, searched everywhere for Tom. She found him in a meeting, grim-faced. Eva announced that she knew Tom would think she was crazy but that Mom, in a dream, had given her a message. Tom was to follow his heart.

Tom hugged her. He had been waiting for that message.

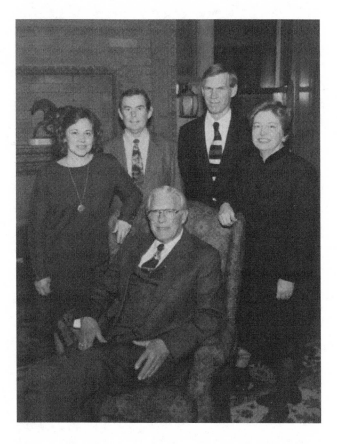

Find Me, Skipper...Promise You'll Find Me

Raised on a horse farm, I experienced nature's wonders. I clucked to the chickens, hatched eggs and fed a milk bottle to deserted lambs. My collie gracefully raced the fields. The following story about Skipper, from its humble author Janine Townsend, lovingly explores our eternal connection with God and beloved animals.

"Skipper was born July 8, 1982 on my farm in Wilmington, OH. I named him Captain Crescent and that was how his name appeared on his Arabian Certificate of Registration. But from the very beginning, I always affectionately called him 'Skipper.'

A long time ago on a warm summer night on my farm in southern Ohio, a newborn foal lay in the soft pasture grass, stretching... waiting...expecting. What he wanted was beyond his reach. But trying hard as he could, his legs simply would not stand up.

As I watched him, I could see something was wrong. I knelt down near him, picked him up in my arms and held him so he could nurse his mother. Somehow during the 11 long months in his mother's womb, his front legs were bent from crowding for space with his twin sister. Sadly, she did not survive, but the little colt did. And from that night on, this little horse and I have shared a very special bond of love.

His one knee would need surgery to help it grow properly and straighten. Many months, casts, bandages and two surgeries later, Skipper grew and learned both horse ways and human ways as we became closer and closer in our relationship. He simply accepted that he had two moms, a four-legged one who nursed him and a two-legged one who fussed over him, and gave him lots of loving.

He was confined to a small paddock and stall until his knee healed and straightened. Finally, he was allowed to venture out with his mother into the big pasture with the other horses. He was quickly relegated to 'last horse' in the herd's pecking order. But to me, he was always 'first.' And he knew it.

Whenever I walked out in the pasture, he would come over and follow me around with his nose softly touching my arm as we walked together. And always, when I would call him from afar, he would answer me. The only times he did not answer my call were times he was in some kind of peril, knowing that his silence would cause me to look for him and rescue him.

He took himself rather seriously and was very persnickety about cleanliness. He avoided anything that would soil his hooves and kept his stall meticulously clean. One corner he reserved for his bathroom. His seriousness about things is what actually made for a lot of comical situations, and so he brought a lot of fun and laughs into our lives.

As the years went by, Skipper has always kept a special place in my heart. Through all of our life's changes that have taken us thousands of miles away from his birthplace, he has always remained an affectionate friend.

We finally settled in Shelbyville, KY in September 2006. By this time, Skipper was 24 years old. While boarding at a neighbor's farm while we were building our own home and barn, he finally found his 'kindred sweetheart' in a big, sweet quarter horse mare, Elvira. The two became so inseparable that it was obvious she would have to become part of our family.

Skipper seemed very content in his retirement years. But in the summer of 2012, he began to develop problems in his hip, which began to interfere with his ability to walk freely and easily. The veterinarian would have to come out every month to give him treatments to help straighten things out, but I was given the warning that this condition would continue to worsen until one day Skipper would no longer be able to get up on his own. I knew that meant that euthanasia was in the future, and that, for me, would be a devastating experience.

A couple of weeks before a strange storm came over our town in late July 2012, Skipper and I were walking in the meadow together. As always, I could feel his nose softly touching my arm as we walked. As I finally approached the fence to get over to our house, I turned to say goodbye for now. But he just stood and stared at me. 'I'll see you tomorrow, Skipper. It's OK. I'll be back.'

Nature can be cruel and merciful at the same time. Just a few weeks after our walk in the meadow, a strange storm began to approach our town. A long black ominous cloud stretched from the west end of Shelbyville all the way east to Bagdad and beyond. But it was strangely flanked on both sides by a cloudless gray sky. My husband and I were at the Lowes in Shelbyville and, noticing this cloud, rushed home to the farm to close windows before the rain began to pour down. Our horses always had free access to the barn from the pasture, but to prevent one getting chased out by the others, I would always put them in stalls during nasty weather.

Upon arriving home, I immediately rushed to the barn to put them in their stalls. At this time of day, which was around five p.m., they generally whinny to see me coming, knowing it must be chowtime. But they were strangely silent. I went into the barn, and looking past the other horses, I could see Skipper oddly staggering to one side. I ran to him and looked in his eyes which were now black and lifeless. 'What's wrong, Skipper, what's wrong?' I ran out of the barn to call the vet, and when I returned, Skipper was laying on the ground. 'Oh, no, not Skipper,' I thought. 'Of all the horses, not him.'

The vet suspected that Skipper had been struck by lightning. As I knelt next to him, he was barely breathing. I stroked him lovingly until his last breath was gone.

My neighbor who has an equine rehabilitation farm across the road from our farm came over awhile later and saw that the marks on his body confirmed that lightning had passed completely through his body. She said he should have been killed immediately. But she believed that he stayed alive just long enough for me to find him and say goodbye. It was the last peril of his life. But this was the final one that I could not rescue him from.

After Skipper passed away I wrote a poem to him, 'Find Me,' asking him to promise me that one day when I pass from this life to the next, that he would come and find me and take me to the place where we all spend our eternity together. Little did I know that Skipper would answer my plea to make this promise.

One late evening in September, while I was working on an online art project, I was watching an artist on YouTube demonstrating how to draw an eye (the window to the soul). While the artist was drawing, there was a beautiful song playing. I was so enraptured by the beautiful song, I had to find out the name of it. I discovered to my surprise that the name of the song was 'Love's Promise.' I began to cry because I knew that Skipper was trying to communicate with me. I went to a website to find the song. And when I found it, he spoke inside my heart to go get his forelock and place it on my poem. (I had saved a little snippet of his forelock before we buried him up on the hill in our meadow.) I got up and found his forelock and brought it back to my poem on my desk. When I went back to the website of the artist, I saw that there was another website I needed to go to next. On the front page of that site was a photo of a very old horse, very heavy set, heavy legs and looking pretty weary. (Skipper by contrast, however, was a very light, and delicate, fine-boned Arabian). This was the moment when he started speaking to my heart. What he said to me gave me comfort about his passing. For in the last few months of his life here on earth, his hip problems were becoming more and more uncomfortable.

His spirit spoke to me: 'This is how I was feeling...so heavy. I didn't want to feel like this anymore.'

Our hearts were together here as we spoke for a while. He wanted me to know it was better for him to be freed from his aging body. I asked him if he was happy and he said yes. I asked him if he would find me, and he told me that he would.

Afterwards, when our conversation was over, I looked up onto the screen where the picture was of the old horse, and there was an image of a forelock! I knew this was his signature that all this really did happen. I held his promise in my heart.

A little more time passed by after this visit with my precious friend, maybe a few weeks or so. I was missing him so very much. One day while at the office, I was searching on my computer for some artwork to use in a marketing piece. I suddenly stopped at a picture of a shadow of a horse standing on a hill far away. As I gazed at the picture, I knew Skipper was somehow wanting to communicate with me again. My spirit was in another place, another realm. As words flowed into my heart, I wrote them down. I shared some of my feelings while writing and the love song was finished. Skipper had answered my plea to him to 'Find Me' and he would keep his promise. This song is 'Skipper's Promise.'

This is how I knew that all of this is real.

The spiritual realm is so very different than what we can ever imagine. The barriers of the physical are gone. Only the spirits remain. There are no barriers to love, to communication, to understanding. Appearances may be no longer as we knew in the physical realm, for no one is any more beautiful than another. Humans and animals may no longer even appear different to each other anymore, for only the spirits remain.

Read the poems and you will experience the bond of love we shared. I will always love him, and miss him, until we are together again."

-Janine Townsend

Find Me, Skipper...Promise Me You'll Find Me

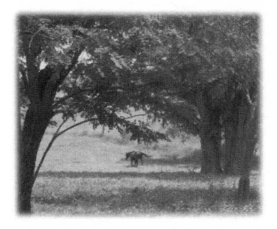

When my body dies in this life
And buried near you on the hill
Promise me you'll find me
Promise me, you will

    Your sweetest whinny whispers
    I'll never hear again
    Your gentle nose upon my elbow
    As we meandered through the glen

        No more calling out your name
        To hear your echoing reply
        So, promise me you'll find me
        Skipper, promise, when I die

            Forever gone in this life
            Faraway upon the hill
            Promise me you'll find me
            Promise me, you will.

            I love you forever, Skipper

Skipper's Promise

My spirit has left the familiar
Searching beyond where I'm needing to be
I see you waiting for me in the distance
Keeping your promise to find me!
I find myself hugging your body
Your mane so silky with light
You're warmth and your love flowing through me
As you carry me with you in flight.
Somehow we are changing together
No bodies, no senses, just eyes
We are the very same spirits together
We now share the very same lives.
The beauty and love so intensified,
And the freedom of spirit released,
You bring me to meet all the others
Such joy beyond all of my dreams!

Surprises

These short vignettes are full of spiritual miracles. A door was opening – what hidden treasures were there?

Mary Ann Moss mentioned it casually, matter-of-factly. After a near-death experience from a car accident, she no longer feared death. As a doctor who had fought for decades to valiantly prevent the tragedy of death, that caught my attention. No longer fear death? How strange, but incredibly fascinating. How much easier life would be without fear? What if patients could be reassured about death? Can we eliminate fear of death by fulfilling our life mission?

Having heard repeatedly about near-death experiences, it had become increasingly clear. They are real phenomena. But what was their meaning? What was their relevance? What could they teach us?

Mary Ann saw a bright light that "did not hurt my eyes, a very beautiful peaceful light. I felt at peace and had joy in my heart that God was in control…I was left feeling that death is nothing to fear, that joy and peace await me." Mary Ann's "knowing" about God is a recurring theme in my patient's experiences. Something special was happening. Something spiritual. Indeed, something that could unlock astounding secrets to the eternal questions we all ponder.

———

Mary Ann's sister-in-law Zoe was boarding the "L-train" in New York City. Suddenly she saw a face identical to her dead mother's. Impulsively, Zoe ran to catch her. As Zoe pushed through the crowds, she lost her. Zoe missed the train. Minutes later the train derailed. All aboard died.

* * * * *

Jack was an alcoholic. In and out of intensive care units for a serious heart condition, he had many close calls. Jack had many regrets about life. He was smart enough, but as the son of a prominent business leader, Jack never lived up to his own high expectations.

During an extended "dry" spell, he married a nice woman and had two fine sons. But alcohol resurfaced. To his great regret, he had abandoned them.

His near-death experience tortured his core being

Without disclosing details, Jack then had a traumatic near-death experience. It shook him up, torturing his core being. Jack stopped drugs. To help his children, he set up trust funds. Jack did everything he could over the next two years to make amends. Then he had another near-death experience. This time it was blissful!

This was the first evidence to me that how you lived your life impacted what transpired at the time of your death. This, for me, was especially transforming. Jack, a smart man, was absolutely changed.

* * * * *

Bonnie heard a clear voice when she was with her 30-year-old brother: "Take care of Charles because his life will be shortened. Always let him know how much you love him." In good health then, Charles died early at age 37.

* * * * *

One night Phil was walking in the woods under the stars. Though an amputee from Vietnam, things were going well.

Suddenly, he was overcome by a presence. Phil could not see it. But it was incredibly powerful. It was unmistakable. He fell to his knees, enveloped by the blissful presence of God.

* * * * *

Cheryl and Carman were traveling together through the Smokies. One morning after they started the day's trip, one of the women uncharacteristically suggested they stop for coffee. They were finishing up when they heard the news. Snipers had shot drivers 10 minutes down the road where they would have been.

* * * * *

Jonathan was having a very painful tooth extraction. Due to his reactions to numbing medicine, no anesthesia was used. Soon, he found himself on the ceiling pain-free, observing.

* * * * *

Delores awoke with a woman in white at the end of her bed. She knew something serious had happened to her daughter Laura. She drove to check on her, knowing Laura did not like unannounced visitors. Laura had just attempted suicide through an overdose.

A woman in white at the end of her bed

* * * * *

A prolonged heart ablation was done for Mira's arrhythmia. When told a second procedure was necessary, she apprehensively prayed. When a third highly intricate procedure was needed, Mira felt vulnerable. Her prayers became urgent. She heard a distinctly audible voice: "I've got it." She knew this was God's voice. Reassured, Mira relaxed. This last procedure "did the trick."

* * * * *

Geri had committed suicide. Years later, Emily awoke with Geri at the end of her bed. She was not transparent, and looked good, with an expression like "here I am."

* * * * *

Melanie had a strong dream premonition that her ex-husband's father would die. She warned her ex Barry to make amends with him. Barry did not follow through. A week later, Barry's father tragically died.

* * * * *

While being treated for a heart attack at the Emergency Department, Daryl had a life-threatening arrhythmia. He left his body and observed from the top of the room. When they shocked him, he went back in body and woke up.

* * * * *

A direct descendent of a Cherokee chief, Martha is from a long line of intuitive people. Martha once saw a dead ancestor. In times of distress, Martha was able to communicate telepathically with her grandmother.

* * * * *

When Amy came to visit, she had an animated, overflowing free spirit. Positive energy poured from her soul. Instantaneously, she read my thoughts to know my reaction to what she said. Amy's facial expressions were extremely sensitive to nuances of my speech.

My mood soared in her presence. She so appreciated the wonderful gifts God had given her. Because of Amy's vulnerability to negative energy, I taught her how to put on an invisible, protective "diamond-studded" body suit.

An invisible protective "diamond-studded" body suit

* * * * *

A week after his father died, Kenneth Hibbs was swinging on his front porch when suddenly he was overcome by the presence of his dead father. It was unequivocal, a reassuring presence that everything was all right. Similarly when at work, Kenneth unmistakably felt the presence of his close friend Mr. Green just days after his death. His message: peace, love and reassurance.

* * * * *

At a subway station, Carla heard the word "suicide." Where did it come from? She was uneasy and immediately began to pray. Then there was a commotion. The next day, she read that a Sam Preston had jumped in front of a subway at the same station, but had been brushed aside. Carla knew her prayers had saved Sam.

* * * * *

Roseanne knows immediately when her son needs her. One night on duty at the hospital she suddenly knew she had to get home to check on her son. She arrived at three a.m. just as her son did, long after he was supposed to be home. Shortly, the police followed him in.

She knows when her son needs her

* * * * *

Pandy stopped progressing with her labor. Medicine helped, but did not last long. Finally, things began happening. Suddenly she found herself next to the ceiling. But within moments she realized, "Hey, I need to have this baby!" She zoomed back into her body.

* * * * *

Rhonda worked with Rachel and had previously met Rachel's mother. Two days after Rachel's mother died unexpectedly, Rhonda walked past Rachel's room at the office. Rachel's mother was sitting in Rhonda's chair.

* * * * *

Though of strong religious faith, Garnetta Bunch had dearly missed her deceased husband Granville. They had been married 60 years before his death. She still longed for his presence.

One morning she awoke from a dream with lips pressing against hers. She immediately recognized the kiss. It was Granville.

* * * * *

One late night Bob, a health practitioner, looked across the room. He saw his friend and simultaneously his three previous lives, one an old man with a beard, another a blond and the third an Indian.

He saw his friend and simultaneously his three previous lives

* * * * *

While being loaded in the ambulance with a severe heart attack, Jose told his brother he would not survive. Jose took what he thought was his last breath. Minutes later, his eyes popped open. In that interval, Jose saw gray with light shining through. It was an incredible state of complete peace and love transformed Jose. "Easily over a thousand" people on three continents were praying for him.

* * * * *

Phil shared that a few days after his grandmother died, she appeared at the foot of his bed. His father reported the identical thing.

* * * * *

Lisa when in college developed strep throat. It evolved into rheumatic fever. She was hospitalized after fainting with a very high blood sugar. Lisa was depressed when a voice said, "Do not be afraid, the Lord is with you." Her blood sugar quickly returned to normal and she was in complete tranquility.

* * * * *

Growing up Tina and her best friend communicated with each other from a distance. Tina did not realize this was unusual. She thought everyone could. She still can sometimes hear others thoughts.

* * * * *

Sharon's surgery was not going well. Unexpected severe bleeding had developed. As she lightly floated upwards, she could see beads of sweat on the surgeon's brow. Sharon captured an ever-larger view of the surgical suite. She hovered as lightly as a feather. She felt complete peace and was enveloped in all-knowing love.

* * * * *

Mike Florence had lost all hope for relieving his back pain. During his third surgery, a metal rod was placed. Mike was bedfast for a year after. On Christmas Eve, he prayed for his life to be taken.

Scripture proclaiming God's immeasurable power gave him inspiration to persevere. He spent an hour nightly reading scripture and another memorizing it. Mike struggled to reduce his addictive narcotic pain medicine. Six months after altering nutrition and starting supplements, his pain was mild requiring only intermittent non-prescription relief. Then over a year he built a church by himself for $30,000, fully donating his labor.

After praying for his life to be taken, he built a church donating his labor

* * * * *

Two-year-old Sawyer had major brain challenges. He was in for his initial patient visit. A charming child, he was easy to examine. Diligently, I worked out a detailed protocol to promote optimal brain growth. Or so I thought.

Sawyer repeatedly tried to get into my handout folders. Despite repeated failures, he finally succeeded in pulling one out. The folder title was "Rhodiola." For Sawyer, Rhodiola would be an outstanding brain-promoting herb, which I had forgotten to consider.

* * * * *

She was performing Reiki on Ginnie, when Gretchen sensed and visualized a large, husky apparition. Without letting on, Ginnie gently described to Gretchen what she was seeing. "Does that sound familiar?" Immediately, Gretchen replied her grandfather, to whom she was very close, was of that description.

Gretchen visualized a large husky apparition

* * * * *

Two days after his grandmother's death, Ron was in his room crying. They were very close. She had cared for him when he was young, and in her final years he was able to repay the attention.

Suddenly Ron felt her presence. As he looked up, she stood before him. "Everything is OK," she reassured him. The two carried on a conversation. Ron's young daughter, peaking through the door, saw it all, though she didn't know to whom her dad was talking.

* * * * *

Pam Warford's mother had the habit of waving frequently; when she passed the door of your room, she always gave a little wave. At burial, the family traditionally releases a balloon with an insignia, which rises in a quick straight path. This insignia was "Love you, Mom." After initially rising, the balloon seemed to hang and began "waving" back and forth. For the next minute, the balloon would not stop waving. The family all knew. This was Mom waving goodbye.

* * * * *

Bethany had recurring severe uterine bleeding. The doctor said she absolutely had to have the uterus removed.

Bethany has had a strong faith since she was three. Her life was forever changed when later baptized. A heavy prayer, Bethany prayed to God to spare her from surgery.

One day at home Bethany heard a voice. "Thank me for healing you." She gushed prayers of Thanksgiving to God. She was healed.

"Thank me for healing you"

* * * * *

Michelle had a dream about how, at her father's funeral, everyone would stand around his casket; when her father died a month later, it was exactly as she had visualized. Michelle communicates with her dead father through a medium. She has seen her father's picture on an orb in the dining room.

* * * * *

For two years after her divorce, Arianne wrangled over visitation. With her children constantly being shuttled back and forth, counselors insisted the children have stability. Arianne gave up primary custody, visiting them every two weeks in Indiana.

One Sunday night after returning them, she fell asleep at the wheel. A voice aroused her. "Wake up Arianne." She had nearly submarined under a semi-truck.

* * * * *

A jolly woman with a big smile, 70-year-old Eleanor has had many spiritual experiences. She has dreams where she sees the interior of houses and feels cozy. Days or months later, she will find herself visiting these houses. They appear just as in her dreams.

Aimee Fulks intuitively can know what is going to happen in advance. This happens commonly, but it is often oddball. Aimee intuited, "A man will enter the room and mention the word 'cherries.'" Within minutes, that very thing happened.

A man will enter the room and mention the word "cherries"

* * * * *

Tim's client Petula had a seizure disorder. After a series of seizures, it was not clear if she would survive. Petula told Tim a very special thing happened during the seizures. In a near-death state, she saw her ancestors. Jesus then told her, "It is not your time."

* * * * *

Dee Dee has always focused on making the world a better place and maintains a special relationship with God. After a diagnosis of ovarian cancer, Dee found herself in an empty room contemplating the meaning. She sent a heartfelt prayer. Though by herself, she clearly heard an audible voice: "You can check out now."

Dee knew then she had a choice. Her heart had given her troubles. She suspected God was offering the option of a quick painless death. Dee Dee had too much to live for. She was not ready to move on.

She then had a stressful time with her family. Her cancer assessment and treatment were anguishing. Dee understands now why God offered to spare her those experiences.

* * * * *

Paul turned 16. He celebrated by swimming in his favorite lake. Diving off a low cliff into murky water, he was stunned by a large tree lying not far under the surface. Paul was drowning.

The water turned a rich, unnatural blue. There was a tunnel behind him he somehow could see. Paul felt at complete peace. Slowly, he turned toward the tunnel. Three girls dove in to save him. Paul has never feared death since.

* * * * *

Angela has always been gifted. One gift, though, she doesn't know how to use. When touched, Angela can tell how soon that person will die.

When touched, she can tell how soon that person will die

Other strange things happen. When standing next to a woman, before that woman knows, Angela can tell if she is pregnant. When having a miscarriage at six months, Angela left her body.

* * * * *

She had a friend who was at Herrington Lake on a Sunday morning. He had been alcoholic. The room was dark. Listening to a Christian radio show he heard, "Who is Jesus? You must decide right now!" He declared out loud, "Jesus, I need to decide now if you are real."

Suddenly the room was infused with rich, comforting warmth. He was overwhelmed. "I think Jesus is my savior, the Son of God." Immediately, the warmth left the room. He was baptized the following Monday morning.

* * * * *

Her husband was highly regarded in her community. At his death, $100,000 was spent on a gravesite in her yard overlooking the community. He had lung cancer and been coughing badly for a year.

On the way to Cracker Barrel, he nearly choked. They turned around, went home and upstairs to bed. The next morning, he came off the elevator saying, "I'll never go back upstairs! An angel visited me saying I was going to heaven."

* * * * *

Barbara's son Jackson had become alcoholic. One day instead of kissing her on the cheek, he surprised her by kissing her on the lips. The next day Jackson became so drunk he passed out, aspirated his vomit and died.

Later, Barbara was at a prayer meeting with other women. She closed her eyes trying to visualize Jesus. Instead, she saw herself as a dancer on the *Lawrence Welk Show*. Suddenly she was dancing with Jesus. Then Jesus turned into her son Jackson. Jackson kissed her on the lips telling her, "It's OK to get well."

* * * * *

Katie's dad, raised a Southern Baptist, had become Buddhist. After her dad died early at age 52, Katie began hearing smoke alarms. The first was when visiting the Shambhala Meditation Center he frequently visited; the fire alarm had never gone off there before. When at home, the smoke alarm spontaneously went off even though there was no smoke. Katie was visiting her father's friend in a nursing home when the alarm went off there. She had a traumatic romantic relationship; as she finished journaling about it, the alarm went off. The night before her wedding near the Red River Gorge area, the alarm also went off.

Alarming communication from beyond

* * * * *

Melissa Dunn Miracle could not cope with the idea that her mother was dying. Melissa was only six. At the hospital she had run out of her mother's room, sobbing uncontrollably.

One night she awoke at three a.m. Unmistakably, Melissa felt the presence of her mother hugging her. It felt so wonderful, so reassuring. Melissa then drifted off to sleep.

Her mother died at six a.m. the next morning. Melissa learned that at three a.m. her mother's heart monitor had flat-lined for two minutes.

A mother's embrace while flat-lined

* * * * *

Shannon had seven miscarriages. She decided to visit Kania, a healer. Energy blockages were identified in Shannon's pelvis. Kania was curious as to what caused them. Shannon shared about her miscarriages. "That explains it," Kania declared. Seven angels surrounded Shannon, one for each chakra, one for each infant.

* * * * *

In 94-year-old Searcy's final days, he became confused, with most conversation incomprehensible. Except for a moment of clarity when his eyes bolted open. Excitedly, he described a white room where he was asked questions, but it was not time yet to answer. He asked them questions, but "it is not yet time for our responses." After this moment of clarity, he resumed babbling.

* * * * *

When Carla was climbing the stairs at a Morehead campus building to have her dissertation reviewed, she heard a loud voice from nowhere. "What is your name?" Intuitively, she stated her name. "What does that name mean?" Her last name, Stephens, means "to witness."

When Carla went into the meeting, one reviewer had been replaced. That professor had been an obstructionist, trying to prevent her graduation. The meeting went beautifully. Carla's thesis topic: "Spirituality and Occupational Medicine."

Afterward, as she was walking down the stairs, Carla saw the obstructionist professor looking up. His mouth was gaping like a five-year-old child, as if something was being revealed.

* * * * *

Middle-aged Catherine had major challenges early in life. I suggested she likely was given a spiritual gift as a result. The topic was dropped until the end of the visit.

"Actually special things have happened," Catherine offered. When her father died, she felt his presence. Distinctly, she felt his hand on her shoulder. She has also felt her mother's presence.

"You may think I'm psychotic, but I see shadows walking around." The house she lives in was the setting for a multiple murder years ago. "I do not care if they visit, but they have to help sweep the house and scrub the floors."

"I do not care if the shadows visit, but they have to help sweep and scrub"

* * * * *

As a high school freshman, Sandra King was in home economics class. Cookies had been burned. The smell permeated the classroom.

Suddenly, Sandra noticed an unusual smell. She asked the other students about it. No, all they sensed were burnt cookies. Sandra knew this was different. She smelled funeral flowers.

The smell of funeral flowers was ominous

Later she learned at that very time her Uncle Steve died in a head-on collision. Uncle Steve had loved her so much. When she had been little, to show Sandra off, he would carry her around everywhere.

Sandra now has stronger premonitions. She develops the urgent need to see particular people. At first she could not understand. Whenever it occurs, she discovered, those individuals died within two weeks.

Sandra once developed a strong urge to see a manager at her work. It was strange in that she did not know him well. The next day he had a seizure and died.

Sandra's role may be to prepare them to move into the beyond. Perhaps it is their last chance to make amends.

* * * * *

Shanna had been abused growing up. She had never wanted to live. In the depths of a depression, she had slit her wrist. Instinctively, she started to call 911. But then stopped.

Shanna was sinking into a coma. A 10-foot tall man with a blue-green coat and black hair appeared. That is the last she remembered.

A 10-foot man with a blue-green coat

Somehow, 911 was called. Shanna thinks the giant applied pressure to her wrist. He saved her life. She is now purpose-driven.

* * * * *

Though slowly dying with cancer, Granddad was not to be kept down, staying active on his small farm. Lynn was talking with sister Carrie when Carrie's six-year-old daughter, playing nearby, suddenly ran up. "Granddaddy is dying! Granddaddy is dying!" "Of course he is Susie, he has cancer." "No! He is dying now!"

A child's intuition saves Granddad

Together they went to check. He was not in or near the house. He was nowhere to be found. Finally, they looked on the farm. His tractor had fallen over, trapping him injured beneath it. He would have died.

* * * * *

The Holocaust and Hitler have always fascinated Cecilia. In college, she majored in German. Her massage therapist Theresa picked up signals from Cecilia's body. Theresa asked her about concentration camps. Cecilia previously died in April 1942 in a concentration camp, Theresa intuited. Her son is an old soul, Theresa sensed, and in a previous life had been her husband.

She previously died in a concentration camp

* * * * *

As a successful businessman, Doug is very disciplined. Many times he has done a three-day pure water fast. The first day is challenging and the second day even more so. On the third day, something spiritual happens. His hunger disappears. Doug hears nearly audible instructions from God about how his life is to proceed. With this clear direction, Doug started a unique, highly successful charity supporting adolescent boys without a home, drawing generous celebrity support.

Connecting to God through fasting

* * * * *

Her minister said it was time to learn to speak in tongues. After visiting him, Mariah began saying a few words in tongues. As her husband drove the family home, Mariah's hands began to burn. Looking down, she could see crosses on her hands burning the skin.

As they continued, Mariah increasingly spoke in tongues. When crossing the threshold of her house, her eyes rolled up. Her appearance was frightening. Fearful, the family quickly scattered.

All of the "negativity" then left her body. When completed, she was cleansed. In essence, Mariah was "reborn." This is "crystallization."

* * * * *

Eva Walter's spiritual church group met with John, the husband of an Episcopalian priest. Incredibly at one point, spiritual stairs appeared next to him.

Spiritual stairs appeared next to him

John died not long afterwards. He had asked that no one share this with his wife, who he knew would not understand.

Eva had a heavy heart and was weak for the next eight months. The priest then came to Eva. She said her husband John had shared spiritually that Eva had something to tell her. With relief, Eva shared the story. Eva's disability quickly resolved.

* * * * *

When her twins were born, Lesa left her body; she was drawn back in when one of the twins cried. Her husband now respects Lesa's intuitions; when he is driving, she will suddenly warn her husband to avoid particular cars.

Her uncle had terminal cancer and Lesa had been assisting in his care. One morning she awoke from sleeping on the couch with her dead grandmother in front of her "as clearly as could be." Her grandmother told her that Lesa's uncle had died. Within minutes a cousin knocked on her door to notify Lesa of her uncle's death.

Her dead grandmother announced his death

* * * * *

Garnetta Graham has had a spiritual connection since childhood. She interacts with two to three angels daily. Gabriel and Michael are amongst them. Each angel has areas of expertise to help her.

Garnetta also has a jaguar that is her guardian animal. She can talk with animals. For example, she can talk to her dog and her dog "talks" back.

* * * * *

A robber was breaking into Missy's house. Immediately, she left her body. Above the ceiling, she could not see her house being pillaged. However, the face of the robber, which Missy had seen briefly, stuck. Later she pointed him out to police.

The experience was so traumatic that Missy stayed out of her body much of the time. One energy healer tried to help, but could not locate her energy field. A healer was finally located and Missy is successfully staying in her body.

* * * * *

On a number of occasions, Sharon had experienced vivid dreams in which she saw people she had never met. That is, until the next day.

She saw people in her vivid dreams she had never met – until the next day

* * * * *

Don's mother had died overnight. He grieved at telling eight-year-old son Junior who had always been so close to his grandmother. Building up his courage that morning, Don tenderly shared the news. "No Dad. Grandmother came to visit me last night. She said everything would be alright." Grandmother visited regularly after that until Junior was 10.

* * * * *

Missy's mother had 15 children. When she died, there was a strong scent of roses. The priest "almost levitated" he was so pleased. This was the affirming "Odor of Sanctity," opposite of a sulfur smell.

"The Lord wakes me up during the night to pray for others. He will say, 'Missy, will you pray for...' One night I was awakened to pray for the Boston bomber while he was being tracked down in a manhunt."

I was awakened to pray for the Boston bomber

* * * * *

Carrie realized she was going to miscarry her pregnancy, but could not convince her doctor. Her husband, accepting the doctor's verdict, tried to reassure her.

After her husband left one day, Carrie laid face down on the couch crying. She prayed out loud that she could not take it anymore. Carrie had to have the Lord's help with this!

A presence arrived. She felt Jesus over her. His hands wrapped around her. Immediately she was reassured. Two days later Carrie miscarried, but she was fine with it.

* * * * *

When she was little, Anita's mother was a dark energy. One day Anita was comforted by an overwhelming loving presence of white entities sparkling like comets.

White entities sparkling like comets

When Anita was 18 and driving to work, she approached her work site. A thought crossed her mind. "Wouldn't it be weird if the two buildings were closed down by a bomb threat?"

As she entered, Anita heard a voice shouting from behind. "Get out immediately! There is a bomb threat. The building has been closed!"

* * * * *

In Toronto, April felt a special presence at a revival. After worshiping for hours, upon approaching the band she walked into an invisible wall and collapsed to the floor. Her friends escorted her to a room. Once there, she felt herself fly to a dark space with a door outlined with a great light. A voice she knew as God's said "You can open the door if you want." She closed her eyes. "One day I will."

Later, she shared the story with some friends, closed her eyes, and in her mind opened that door. A bolt of light flashed. Those in the room held out their hands. It was raining mercy.

A bolt of light flashed...It was raining mercy

* * * * *

Patty Holtman has premonitions about people in need. When 11 years old, Patty had recurring dreams of falling, awakening her in a panic. When she asked her mother, "Where will I go when I die?" she was sent back to bed. When grown, needing to know if she was saved, Patty got on her knees and closed her eyes. Patty literally saw Jesus on the cross. He told her, "If you were the only one in the world, I would still go to the cross for you." She cried and asked for forgiveness. When praying about when her husband would be saved she was told, "It will be cold outside, but in your husband's heart it will be spring time." He was saved in November

* * * * *

"While dropping my son off, I saw from the corner of my eye a giant bear in front of a church across the street. When I did a double take, the bear of course was no longer there, but I had seen it. Later I got a call from school that my son was in trouble. In a dream book, the bear symbolized 'some misfortune.' My son was later expelled.

While looking in the bathroom mirror, a fly landed on the corner of my eye. When I opened my eye after blinking, my eye was completely bloodshot. When I blinked again, my eyes were normal. Minutes later, my daughter comes in crying. Her cousin accidentally poked her in the eye while playing basketball and her eye was completely bloodshot."

-Kelly Shepherd

* * * * *

Anne Hopkin's job at Good Foods Coop had become very stressful. One night, she suddenly sat up in bed. A voice distinctly said, "Your name is Soaring Spirit. You do not have to be afraid."

"Your name is Soaring Spirit. You do not have to be afraid."

She has been relaxed ever since and is retiring to her farm to grow organic vegetables and start Broody Hill Farm Bed and Breakfast next to Lake Cumberland.

* * * * *

While pregnant, Lena developed a blood clot in her leg. She was very ill, as she was medivaced out of Ecuador. Her predeceased grandfather, who she had been close to, came to tell her, "It is not your time. You are OK. You can relax now." Lena recovered.

Since, she has become intuitive and sensitive to negative energy. Three psychics on different continents upon learning her age of 40 commented her real age, her spiritual age, was 21. That is the number of years since her near-death experience.

* * * * *

Margaret entered a bar and saw a man across the room. A voice said,

"That's the man you will marry."

"That's the man you will marry"

She looked around. There was no one who could have said that. Margaret and Jon have been married now for 20 years.

* * * * *

Ramona, who has left her body on several occasions, may have been saved by a premonition. Riding "shotgun" in a friend's car, Ramona suddenly shouted to her friend, "Pull over, pull over!" They came to a stop. Her friend, Ramona knew, had to be having strange thoughts. Just then, a truck came barreling over the hill in the wrong lane.

* * * * *

Mary was a close friend of Lydia's in high school. Then a car accident tragically ended Mary's life. They had shared so many memories together. Mary was always there for her. Lydia, overcome with sadness, cried inconsolably.

Suddenly, an angel appeared. Lydia could feel the love emanating from this celestial being. Immediately, she felt at peace.

* * * * *

Kim and her four-year-old son riding next to her were broadsided on his side. The car smashed completely up against her. Kim was horrified because she could not feel her son and knew he must have been crushed. She cried uncontrollably when she felt a hand tap her on the shoulder. Somehow, her son was in the backseat. "Mommy, an angel carried me to the back seat."

"Mommy, an angel carried me to the back seat"

* * * * *

"I was home alone, wide-awake, sitting at a laptop computer. Suddenly, I glanced up and 'saw' Dr. Charles sitting on the futon, with his head turned toward me. I was startled and turned my head to the left. I saw the same vision.

Dr. Charles appeared as if posing for a portrait, he looked younger than he was when we met in 1963. He was wearing dark-rimmed glasses, and his head was slightly turned so his right ear was more prominent. He had a closed mouth smile. I grabbed a scrap of paper and sketched his facial expression with a pencil. No words were spoken. I accepted his visit as an encouragement to continue studying energy medicine as a way to maintain my health."

An after death visit from her boss

-Sunny Churchill

* * * * *

Maureen, feeling challenged, one evening heard fireworks. When she looked out the window, a cloud was shaped like an angel. She felt a calming presence. Everything would be OK.

A friend saw her dead alcoholic husband walking, as he always did, to the library with a cane, glasses near the edge of his nose. On double take, he was still there. On a third glance, he looked her straight in the eyes. His voice said, "Tell Maureen I'm sorry."

———

She has always wanted to be a missionary. At her new husband's church, the missionary speaking asked if there was a Maureen in the audience. Maureen thought he was confusing her with Charlene in front of her, but her other family members heard. Afterwards, she introduced herself to the missionary. He was stunned, as he had no recollection, or reason to say, this.

* * * * *

They lived 50 miles from the nearest house in the far northern reaches. Periodically, Selena Brinson and her mother would see UFOs – metallic discs in the sky that sometimes hovered for days.

Selena and her mother would see UFOs

One night when they were driving home it was extremely dark. A light appeared in the distant sky that kept getting brighter. The next thing they knew, she and her mother were home and had missed two and a half hours. Since that moment, Selena has been more intuitive.

As an acupuncturist at Wellspring Massage Therapy, Selena studies continuously. She is intent on being the best. When placing needles, Selena can often intuit her patient's issues. She can then counsel them. When her needle hits the problematic spot, Selena feels a surge of electrical energy and her hands begin to shake.

* * * * *

Alisha was delivering her baby who had anencephaly, a deformity where the top of the brain is missing. She was given a drug to knock her out during delivery.

Alisha floated to the ceiling while the baby was dying during childbirth. She asked the doctor repeatedly how her baby was doing, but he of course could not hear her. While out of body still, she then met her baby, now six years old and with a full beautiful head. This put her at complete peace. There was no post-traumatic stress.

* * * * *

Carrie had a strong premonition. Something bad was about to happen. Through past experience, she had learned to pay attention. The next day, Carrie knew she had to stay home. Then at the front door and at the back door simultaneously, two men were trying to break into her house. Carrie was prepared. She frightened them. They scattered.

An Astonishing Conference

Experiences of Health Practitioners early in my journey were incredulous. A whole new world was unfolding. An integrative cancer movement, inspired and rooted in the genius former-monk Donald Yance, and catapulted by the brilliant integrative oncologist Dwight McKee, served as the setting for these profound experiences.

In the spring of 2013, my exploration bore new fruit. Health colleagues at an integrative cancer conference in Arizona shared amazing, perplexing and inspiring encounters.

A strawberry blond, Dr. Ann Ross boasted distinctive glasses and a feisty personality. An older physician from the Northwest, she confided that periodically her dead Aunt Rosie spoke to her.

The messages were not earthshaking. But Ann thought it odd that she frequently heard this voice. Finally she dismissed the thoughts, telling herself, "Well, that's just like Aunt Rosie!"

Odder still was a familiar male's voice invading Ann's head, a voice from the past, one she had not invited. Ann specifically disliked and distrusted this voice. But it frequently returned. The voice was very insistent. Ann must take a message to her niece Melissa.

Bill was engaged to marry Melissa. Dr. Ross did not find him a particularly impressive suitor. She was not happy about their plans. Two weeks before they were to get married, Bill committed suicide. Melissa was distraught. She could not understand.

Bill, now in another realm, was restless. He had to let Melissa know why. Across that impenetrable veil, Bill still loved her dearly.

To dispel the annoying, disruptive voice, Ann relented. She shared with Melissa the story Bill had coached her to share.

Across that impenetrable veil, Bill still loved her very much

For Melissa, it was an answer to her prayers. She so wanted to know why. Bill had reached across from the other side. He had given her answers. Most importantly, he expressed his love was for all time.

* * * * *

Hallie, a highly regarded digestive expert, was traveling on the Washington, D.C. beltway with her toddler son. Peter, recently having turned two, was snuggly buckled in his car seat. Ahead loomed the beltway's single tall hill. As they started the long climb, a Mercedes cruised just ahead in the left lane. Rush hour traffic moved them along hurriedly.

Suddenly a voice spoke to Hallie. "Get in the right lane!"

No one else was in the car. Never had she heard voices. Hallie was confused. Was she hallucinating? She must have imagined it. Then the voice bellowed louder, this time commanding, insistent and urgent, "Get in the right lane!"

Hallie switched lanes as they crested the hill. Just on the other side in the left lane, the Mercedes was careening off of a semi-truck.

* * * * *

Julia picked up dinner at the restaurant counter. She then located a secluded spot to collect her thoughts.

A man approached, pointing his finger at her. Emphatically, he stated, "You are blessed!"

Over the following month, she was not herself. Odd things would happen. Julia was afraid that if asked to speak she would have no voice.

Suddenly, she heard a voice offering an explanation. Its message was a surprise. The angels "wanted to dress her up." Julia was clueless as to what that meant.

The voice identified itself. It was her spiritual guide, Ezekiel. He had come to her on her 30th birthday, April 5th.

After this pronouncement, Julia ran to her Bible. Hurriedly, she opened to the book of Ezekiel. The first line shook her world.

"Now it came to pass in the 30th year, in the fourth month, on the fifth day…that the heavens were opened and I saw visions of God."

"…It came to pass in the 30th year, in the fourth month, on the fifth day"

From time to time, Ezekiel returns, offering sage advice.

* * * * *

Denise and her husband Jack were moving to the west coast. They had left their children with close friends near their new home. On their way to Omaha, Denise had foreboding thoughts. A frightening, recurring mental image emerged – a lifeless body floating in water.

On entering their motel room, they were shocked. A tall man was on their bed. Startled, he jumped up. As he bolted between them in the doorway, he brushed against their shoulders. Turning down the hallway, Denise and Jack both witnessed it – the man disappeared. The message then arrived. Their two-year-old James had been in a drowning accident. His friend had alerted his parents that James was at the bottom of the pool. Motionless and blue, he was pulled out. Rescuers performed CPR for two hours before he responded. James was left in a coma. When word got out, many were praying for him.

When Denise and Jack arrived early the next morning, James later shared he knew it was time to wake from his coma. Doctors told

Denise her son would unavoidably have major brain damage. Despite this ominous warning, in 24 hours James' brain had "reset." Except for a short-lived limp, he was back to normal.

"Was James different after that?" I inquired. "Oh yes. He has a very strong spirituality." When the parents of a neighborhood family died suddenly, they adopted one of the four children. The other three got into trouble, one on drugs. But Jarred, whom they adopted, was now well-adjusted and productive thanks to James' influence.

James, a successful nurse practitioner, said as a child his soul would leave his body. It traveled to many areas around the country. He could see these communities very clearly.

As a child his soul would leave his body and travel to many areas

Later, when the family was on trips, he would recognize communities he had visited earlier. It turned out these were communities with a church that had prayed for James when he was in a coma. Churches in both hemispheres of the Americas had prayed for James.

A year after the drowning incident, a business firm in a nearby city hired Jack. It turned out the CEO of that large business was a member of a church praying for their son. Though not there physically, this was the same startled man in their motel bed.

* * * * *

Jana, a nurse, was flying with Cheryl, her one-year-old baby. Jana was packing baby items in her luggage when Cheryl began vomiting. Jana had to make a connecting flight at the Boston airport, which she knew to be a complex task. Jana fretted. How was she going to make it with a vomiting baby?

Upon arriving at the Boston airport, they rushed into the terminal. A man asked very nicely if they needed help. He guided Jana with baby in tow through the airport, assisting with her baggage.

After nearly reaching her departure gate, Jana was briefly distracted. When turning back to thank her assistant, he was nowhere to be seen. It was at a junction of two hallways. She could see clearly down both hallways. There was not a trace of this man.

* * * * *

Nat, a naturopath, is a warm, spiritual conversationalist. Four years earlier, she had developed melanoma. It advanced to its end stage. Nat researched integrative approaches thoroughly. She also connected spiritually in a profound way.

Nat has been healed. She has developed many successful integrative strategies. New intuitive abilities have helped her heal many in need.

* * * * *

As a child Erin had been playing with her friends. In a nearly finished house, they found a new refrigerator. Who could stay the longest inside it?

When it was her turn, she climbed in. When a parade arrived in front of the house her friends, distracted, ran to watch.

It was very dark in the refrigerator. She could not get out. It was getting frigid. As time passed she became very frightened.

Finally, the door opened. A very small man pleasantly greeted her. It was a leprechaun. Then he vanished.

Phenomenal Mystery and Magnificence

The brilliance and radiance of these experiences became an obsession. No longer satisfied, I had to know more.

A spiritual woman, Darlene lamented that her son joined the armed forces. She knew, though, she had to let go. Perry joined a special fighting unit reflecting a good mind and strong determination. Training was going well. But many vigorous soldiers struggled through the swim test. Perry had to swim a long distance underwater.

When police came to her house, they avoided eye contact. Having lost an infant after birth, Darlene knew what it meant.

Darlene prayed vigorously. She had studied prayer intently. From a detailed prayer book, she learned exactly how to pray. Darlene told God that while Perry had not been the best person, he had much life to live. God needed to spare his life.

When she got to the hospital, they told Darlene he was not responding to CPR. She continued praying vigorously. Suddenly, Perry's eyes jolted open.

Doctors told Darlene he would have major brain damage. Within two weeks, Perry was riding a bicycle. He had a complete recovery. She knew without a doubt prayer had spared his life. His doctor later told Darlene that Perry was not supposed to survive. His serum potassium level had dropped to one, incompatible with life.

* * * * *

A spiritual mental-health worker believes schizophrenic hallucinations are at times real, connecting into another realm. While at first this seemed outlandish, it has been fascinating to contemplate.

Regina, a bipolar patient, experienced a psychotic episode when smoking marijuana laced with unknown drugs. Soon afterwards, she felt flames lapping against the underside of her thighs, lasting 20 minutes. She had little doubt as to what this experience represented.

In the decades since, she has had a fear of hell. As a devout conservative Southern Baptist, Regina is compelled to repent daily. That a 66-year-old would be anxious about this for decades was an eye opener, and a unique, wonderful opportunity for healing.

While most who are resuscitated do not recall having a near-death experience, those who had an experience generally recall a blissful, spiritual one. In his book *Erasing Death*, Sam Parnia, M.D. found that most who attempt suicide have negative near-death experiences.

Most who attempt suicide have negative near-death experiences

Dr. Parnia's work mirrors my experience, where 98 percent of those who share a clear recollection have felt overwhelming peace and love. My one exception was Jack, who after transforming his life reversed his frightening experience.

As Dr. Parnia noted, 80 percent who have a brush with death do not recall any experience. What would be their fate? Are these among the ones my patients report have not transitioned?

Did Regina experience a taste of the negative future that a life of drugs would produce? How often are negative experiences simply the summation of a life review? Regina could control her future. A discussion of spirituality ensued, which she found reassuring.

* * * * *

Shelia at nine years old was on vacation with the family at a lake in

Arkansas. As they swam, older children took off their life jackets, so Shelia did too. She was dog paddling when Shelia suddenly realized how far from shore speedboat waves had pushed her.

She panicked. Shelia struggled for air as her chest filled with water. She had a life review, recalling many pleasant things from her life. Shelia felt guilty because her parents had spent so much on her braces and she would not survive to take advantage of them.

She took a deep breath. Then everything seemed fine. This made no sense because Shelia knew she was drowning.

She looked down and couldn't find her arms or her legs. Below was a straggle-haired girl face down in the water. Shelia saw in the distance all of her family and relatives standing on the beach horrified.

Below was a straggle-haired girl face down in the water

Shelia saw her aunt kick off her cork-heeled shoes. Shelia asked God, "Tell Aunt Sharon it is OK." She heard, "It is going to be OK." She watched her aunt reach the little girl floating in the water.

Shelia told God, "I do not want to leave Mom and Dad!" But she liked how she felt, completely whole. She was reassured that she was "completely OK." She was "in the light" with wonderful music similar to a Gregorian chant. She was not scared and wanted to hold onto that feeling. Shelia sensed humans are too wrapped up in rules. God is about relationships.

Something jerked her back down, and when pulled to shore, she was ashen. Her pediatrician uncle pumped the water from her chest.

* * * * *

Her daughter Lena was on drugs. Helen prayed. It was Saturday night. On Monday, Lena was to enter a hospital program. She overheard her daughter mention "party" on the phone.

The year before, Lena had been riding with a drunken driver. A serious wreck ensued with Lena fracturing her leg

Now, while riding with her boyfriend Tom, Lena had a premonition about Satan. Her boyfriend reassured her there was nothing to worry about. Words strangely flowed from her mouth: "You are no more than a little worm to Satan that he can easily crush."

"You are no more than a little worm to Satan that he can easily crush"

Meanwhile, Helen had major foreboding. She immediately stopped what she was doing and rushed home. "The Lord gave me a prayer," Helen relayed. "Father build a shield, open her mind and protect her." Opening her Bible, Helen read, "For this child I have prayed and God hath given me petition." She went to sleep reassured.

Suddenly she awoke. It was midnight. Her daughter Lena stood before her wild-eyed.

Lena and her boyfriend had stopped to pick up a friend for the party. Suddenly, Lena saw blood. Helen had taught, "When in doubt, ask God." "Tom, if I go to the party, I will return in an ambulance or a coffin!" Lena and Tom skipped the party to play cards at her friend's house.

"…If I go to the party, I will return in an ambulance or coffin!"

"God spoke those words through me!" Lena exclaimed to her Mom.

At two a.m., Helen was listening to the air conditioner. The sound rose into a strong wind. It transformed into quadraphonic, ethereal voices. It was the perfect choir. She still recalls the melody.

When the two arrived at the hospital Monday, Lena refused drugs for withdrawal. When she had no withdrawal symptoms, the doctor accused her of lying. Days passed. Lena was dismissed.

* * * * *

Karen had always been intuitive. She could recite what was going to be said during a phone call before the phone rang.

Karen's daughter Amanda married in her late teens. After experiencing abuse from her husband, Amanda committed suicide.

Two weeks before, when she was in a quiet place, Karen heard God's voice telling her, "Amanda isn't going to be with you for long." Karen intuited the feeling from the book of Job.

"Will she be here for college graduation?" "No."

"Will I get to watch her get married?" "No."

"Will she be alive in six months?" "No."

"Will she be alive in three months?" "No Julie, it will not be long."

After her daughter died, Karen no longer wanted to be intuitive. She prayed that the intuition be taken away. It has been.

GOD: "Amanda isn't going to be with you for long"

* * * * *

Martha's two-year-old son Johnny one afternoon somehow managed to dislodge the "fence" at the top of the stairs.

Realizing what had happened, Martha panicked. She reached the stairs just as Johnny began a rapid tumble. Martha did not want to grab an arm, knowing that would alter his tumble in an awkward way, increasing fracture risk. Frighteningly, at the bottom of the stairs was a stone landing.

Near the bottom of the stairs Johnny's tumble dramatically slowed. Miraculously, he gently landed sitting on the next to last stair.

Months later Johnny revealed, "Mommy, remember the time I fell down the stairs? My guardian angel caught me and sat me down."

* * * * *

When she was six-years old, Lela's parents divorced. She and her mother moved in with Grandma, sleeping together upstairs in a storage room.

One night Lela saw ghouls, one with a knife. She was terrified. Her mother, of strong Catholic background, said these might be demons. She counseled her to be very good.

Later as an adult, Lela talked with a neighbor about the house. "Oh yes!" the neighbor responded. "That house is haunted!"

Before Lela met her second husband Sam, he had been previously married. His wife June, when dying, at times was delirious. She repeatedly pleaded, "Keep that woman away!"

Later, Lela was at a dinner party. It was before she knew Sam well. A woman was being clearly flirtatious with Sam. Lela was overcome by the presence of Sam's first wife June, who communicated that the "woman" was after her husband! She pled with Lela, "Keep Sam from marrying her!"

Lela was overcome with the presence of Sam's first wife

Lela successfully intervened. And of course married Sam herself.

* * * * *

Melissa Worrell never read the Irvine paper, but when on an errand in town, she happened to glance at it. An ad caught her eye. Contents of a daycare center were for sale. Melissa was overcome by an encompassing, exhilarating, loving presence. It powerfully confirmed what her mind was saying. "OK, OK." Her husband, who had joined her, was perplexed. "What's that about?!" That led to a successful, gratifying business. Melissa was providing a community service she knew was desperately needed.

Melissa once awoke sensing herself levitating. Rising higher, she could see 360 degrees – every direction at once.

A young three-year-old niece once overheard Melissa's conversation about the niece's grandfather who had died before she was born. "He's OK," her little voice softly said. "He comes to see me."

Melissa's father Ted had been at Vietnam. Near the end of his life, war disabilities landed him in the Veteran's Hospital. Once, Ted nearly died. As he lost consciousness, Ted descended into a deep darkness. Grittily, he clawed his way out. Ted recognized his brush with death foretold a destiny he wanted to desperately avoid. He was transformed. From that moment, Ted joyfully brightened the lives of all around him.

Ted descended into a deep darkness

* * * * *

She lost her beloved blind cat, Helen Keller. Afterwards, Carla couldn't contemplate a new cat. But a year later she visited the pound. Of course, just to see the pets, most certainly not to get one.

When Carla and the keeper entered, all of the cats were very serene except one longhaired black and white tuxedo that tore around the cage. It did acrobatics to capture attention. Carla decided to let it out.

It sprinted free, scampering around the room and bouncing off the walls as if to say, "Take me, take me." Of course she did.

When home, "Mariah" sprinkled in the sink. Carla was upset until she realized how smart that was. Thereafter, Mariah always tinkled at the tub drain and pooped at the other end. Carla never needed kitty litter.

When Mariah became old, a butterfly visited, landing on Carla's hand. It walked up to her shoulder, staying there for two hours while she did yard chores. Later, inside, she left the butterfly on the sofa.

A butterfly stayed on her shoulder for two hours while she did yard work

Then, simultaneously, Mariah and the butterfly died. For the next two days outdoors, Carla felt Mariah's strong presence.

* * * * *

Catherine was the proud mother of two daughters, Shelia, age 16, and Brenda, age 13. While Catherine was riding with her husband to Louisville, Shelia was at home looking after Brenda.

Suddenly, Catherine developed an uneasy feeling about her daughters. She immediately called home. There was no answer so she left a message that she was checking on them and was worried about them. After a glance at her watch, Catherine commented on the answering machine that she now remembered they were not due home for another 10 minutes.

At the time she called, there was a robber in the house. He had left permanent tracks on the carpet all over the house, had stolen their computer and even taken items like baby teeth. Catherine felt certain the answering machine message had rushed the robber out of the house. If she had not called, her daughters would have walked in on the robber. Nothing good would have come of that.

The robber even took baby teeth

* * * * *

"I was 29 years old with children ages one and two, and had been dealing with Crohn's disease for two years. My husband was very controlling, abusive to my children and me, and knew which buttons to push to activate the Crohn's disease. Neither of us was happy.

I became very depressed and wondered what I would do about this. One night I was sleeping, and all of a sudden I was floating up in the corner of our bedroom. I could see both of us sleeping on the bed.

The next thing I knew, I was in a black tunnel and there was a light at the end of it. The feeling I had was peace beyond belief! There really aren't any words to put to that feeling of awesome peace!

As I was getting closer to the light, I was arguing with God. I told Him I could not leave my babies yet. I could not bear the thought of them having to live with their abusive father. But I also wanted to continue toward the light. It was so wonderful, peaceful and loving! It was an extremely hard decision to make. Needless to say, God let me return.

I was arguing with GOD

After that wonderful experience, my intuition and discernment are much stronger. I can feel negative energy and danger. I can also see God's light in people, and they can see His light in me. My faith and trust in God has become much stronger! This experience gave me the strength to leave and divorce my husband. God is always in control and guiding us. His love for us is extremely strong!"

-Deborah Shellenberger

* * * * *

"My grandparents lived in a small town in Kentucky, and back during World War I they used to invite the headmaster of the local Presbyterian Academy, a bachelor, for Sunday lunch and to spend the afternoon. After lunch, the three of them would sit in front of the fire and talk. One of the topics they used to discuss was whether or not there was a spiritual world. Eventually the headmaster was called away to the war, and he told them that if he were killed in the war, he would try to come back and communicate with them somehow.

Sure enough he was killed, and the first Sunday after he was killed, my grandparents began to hear this loud rapping on the glass doors of the bookshelves that stood on each side of the fireplace where they used to talk with the headmaster. They described the rapping as hard enough that it seemed like the glass would break, and this would take place every Sunday afternoon for one year to the day.

His ghost returned after the war

Then the rapping stopped and was never heard again."

-John Roach

* * * * *

When arriving home, Rosa Johnson felt fine. But when entering the kitchen she noticed fog setting in. As she walked down the hall, the fog worsened. At one point she was unable to see. She told herself, "Keep going, keep going."

Rosa made it to her bed and climbed in. Through the fog, she could see a vague figure. Then a voice.

"Everything is OK, everything is OK, everything is OK. I'm right here with you, I'm right here with you. Rest my child." The voice reassured Rosa. In fact, she felt "marvelous."

Five minutes later, she realized. No one was there. Except God.

Rosa drifted to sleep. On awakening, everything was back to normal. Rosa learned from this to stop worrying.

The night Rosa shared her story followed a minor confrontation I had at work. My blood pressure I am certain was high. It was hard to focus on anything else. After Rosa shared her story, I completely relaxed.

It is very unusual for Rosa to stop by the office with her husband, who comes nightly. For some reason beyond consciousness, she came. It is my belief she came because her story needed to be shared, and I needed to hear it.

Rosa had only shared her story with two others. She had not told her husband because he "did not believe such things."

Her husband "did not believe such things"

* * * * *

Marsha's dead mother came to her in a "cloud" saying, "I love you." In less than a week, Marsha was admitted to the hospital. Her dialysis port was failing. But things worked out. Surgery was not necessary. Marsha felt her mother was offering her advanced reassurance.

Marsha dreamt that her son was in the hospital with an IV. She told her son, who joked about it. A week later, he had to go to the hospital for an illness requiring an IV.

While having gallbladder surgery, Marsha left her body, watching it all from above.

Marsha was sleeping one night when she woke up with something strangling her. She then sensed her spirit leave her body and combat a demonic spirit back and forth across the ceiling. She finally was able to get to a window, open it and say "In the name of Jesus, demon be gone." She now routinely sweeps evil spirits out of her house.

When she shared this with her husband, he laughed. Until he woke one morning being physically strangled. He no longer laughs.

He laughed…until it happened to him

* * * * *

Genia was very close to her Aunt Mary. Aunt Mary always began each conversation with "Darling…"

When Aunt May was hospitalized with a severe illness, Genia asked if there was anything she could do. "Yes, I would like some dark skinned grapes." Genia went all over town, but could not find any. She had to leave town to find them. When she returned, Aunt Mary had died. She realized Aunt Mary did this so she would not be there when she died.

Two mornings later the phone rang as she awoke. Genia answered.

"Darling,.."

"Aunt Mary, is that you?"

"Yes, darling, I'm in heaven. It is wonderful here!"

"I'm in heaven. It is wonderful here"

She named all the ancestors she had seen. Genia had many more questions, but the dial tone interrupted.

———

Genia's grandson Jim had major emotional issues. No one knew how to help. Growing up, Jim had never gotten help or emotional support from his biological father Jared. When Jared died, Genia prayed to Jared, saying he had not done his job. He needed to help Jim.

Suddenly Jim's mental health turned around. Relatives asked repeatedly, "What happened to Jim that he has improved so much?"

* * * * *

Winnie's daughter Melinda died at 16.

A year later, Winnie awoke paralyzed. She felt the wind blow through her right shoulder, exiting her left hip. She had a knowing beyond all doubt it was her daughter. In those moments, she was transformed.

In a vivid twilight dream, she went to a place of all knowing. There Winnie knew everything she ever wanted to know. As she awakened Winnie became fearful she was going to forget all of the great knowledge she had learned.

Indeed, her knowledge did begin to fade. Winnie asked to be able to remember it all. She was told that, while she would not remember it all, there were just two things she needed to remember. The first was "Love." The second was "Connect to the Light."

Just two things to remember: "Love" and "Connect to the Light"

When Winnie said she was just waiting to die, she was corrected. "No. You are preparing to die. From the day you were born, you have been preparing to die."

———

Winnie later dreamt about three children and their mom. One, a boy, came into full view. Winnie sensed he was dead. Looking her in the eye he offered, "I know you are asking about your daughter. She is fine." Winnie was sure he was referring to her precious Melinda.

Winnie asked, "Are the streets of heaven paved with gold?" "Yes," he said, "and they are so smooth you can drive just as fast as you want!"

At church, she started a conversation with Tara whose son had also died in his mid-teens. Tara also had two other sons, both living. Winnie sighed. "I wonder where my deceased daughter Melinda is."

Tara smiled. "She is with Davy." Davy was the name of the dead boy in Winnie's dream. She asked to see a picture of Davy. The picture of this boy in his mid-teens looked similar to Davy.

The mother then pulled out a picture from when Davy was nine. It was a dead-ringer. He was the Davy she had met in her dream.

"It was a dead-ringer…the Davy she had met in her dream"

———

Another dream at twilight found Winnie levitating above her bed with lights all around. For Winnie, it was like a communion. She had an incredible sense of ecstasy. "I hesitate to share it in this way," she told me, "but I was having an orgasm with every single cell in my body!"

———

Winnie's husband, when dying, was able to read minds. His daughter sleeping next to him in bed had a dream. In the dream, she asked him a question. She awoke suddenly. He was answering the question in person.

At the end, Winnie could communicate with her husband telepathically.

* * * * * *

Sharie was a generous Christian woman. But when diagnosed with ovarian cancer, she stopped praying. Daily she suffered, but did not pray. She felt abandoned by Christ. When her condition deteriorated, she was hospitalized. Sharie's roommate also had advanced cancer.

Once while there, Sharie's spirit rose from her body. As she looked down, she saw the form of Christ pass by. Jesus asked her, "Are you ready to recognize me and be healed?"

Sharie was afraid. She thought if Jesus saved her that her roommate would die. Christ repeated: "Are you ready to recognize me and be healed?"

"Are you ready to recognize me and be healed?"

She hesitated. Then she blurted out, "Yes, I am ready to be healed!" Sharie went back in her body and had a full recovery.

* * * * *

Justin Taylor knew death was certain. Having enlisted for Afghanistan, he always understood the moment might come. And he had volunteered for a risky special mission.

As he watched a shell land in front of him, Justin knew death was imminent. He covered his face with his hands so his parents would recognize him. Within a split second, Justin had a life review. Everything in his entire life, good and bad, passed before his eyes, greatly tinged with emotion. Somehow, and he does not understand why, he was not hurt.

Months later during the war, he was sitting with a buddy. For no reason, he got up and left. Almost immediately a mortar exploded at that spot.

* * * * *

Carmen Allende and husband Jonathan were visiting Boston, cross-country from their home in Phoenix. In church, when her eyes closed, Carmen experienced a powerful vision of a house. She opened her eyes and it disappeared. But it reappeared when she closed them.

For affirmation of this vision, she asked for signs. For her, two important ones were doves and roses. Intriguingly, everywhere she went she now saw doves and roses.

After sharing her vision, she asked Jonathan if they could give up their jobs in Phoenix and move to Boston. He replied he had not seen a vision. She was nuts!

"...He had not seen a vision. She was nuts!"

She reminded him when you marry, two become one. Not fully convinced, but revering his wife, he agreed. Jonathan had learned to trust her intuition. They both gave up their jobs and were set to move. Scouring Boston, however, they could not find a place to call home. A day was set to decide.

On the final day, Carmen told her sister Ouita she had given up. She was worn out. It was time to stop looking. Ouita insisted otherwise. They began a final trek through town. But at the end of the day, nothing had appeared.

They turned to go home when something caught Carmen's eye. Her eyes widened. Was it the house in her vision? Carmen remembered that special house had chocolate doors. But it was dusk. She could not quite see. Carmen and Ouita tore through the yard. When they saw the chocolate doors, they screamed!

When they saw the chocolate doors, they screamed!

For the next 11 wonderful years, Carmen and Jonathan lived in that Boston home, the home of their destiny.

* * * * *

Savannah had a blissful near-death experience, but was told this was the last of three chances she had been given. Growing up she was challenged by an unforgiving mother. At age five she developed psychic insights. Ghoulish figures would arise from the floor.

Harper, a husky fellow in a Harley jacket, having heard of her psychic abilities, approached Savannah. "I think you have a message for me."

Someone was missing in his life. This she could tell. Someone younger. Was it Harper's son?

"My son Jim Owen died in a car accident when 18 years old. He had been at a bar drinking with friends. The others had left. He was seen exiting the bar at four a.m. His wrecked car was found on the side of the road."

Savannah and Harper decided to drive that fatal road. Soon they approached the tree Harper's son had hit. Curious, she asked if a deer had jumped in front of the car. Harper grunted, "I'm sure that was not it." Savannah was unconvinced. "Why are you so sure?" As they reached that spot in the road, three deer crossed.

Savannah said, "He died on his birthday." Harper replied, "Yes, that is true." She saw a sequence. "Chink, chink, chink." Harper looked up surprised. His birthday was 5/5/05.

Savannah saw another chink, chink, chink. "Another special event was 7/7/07. That was the day his dog Pat died. My son cried and cried." He had an elaborate funeral attended by neighborhood kids. He vowed to Pat he would never forget him. He memorialized that date.

Harper could no longer hold back. She had clearly made a connection. "Is there a message from my son? Be sure to tell him that I love him!"

"Yes, he says he loves you, too." Harper began sobbing.

"Yes, he says he loves you too"

———

When Savannah's boyfriend had injuries, she offered to heal them. He resisted. But when a contact lens scraped his eye, he called her. Her left eye began watering. "Yes, it is my left eye," he said. With her healing connection, within minutes he was well.

* * * * *

Elane Moore was six years old when her school principal in Barbourville, West Virginia died. Elane overheard her mother and a neighbor talking about his death. The conversation shifted to whether there was an afterlife. Elane was shocked. She assumed everyone knew for certain about God and the afterlife. She has known her whole life.

Elane's first memory was prior to her birth. It was of luminous white shimmering gowns flowing back and forth that she could see only from the waist down. They were saying, "You volunteered for this project." She replied, "But I changed my mind." She heard, "It is too late." Then with a shove, she remembers being pushed into her new existence.

Elane's first memory was prior to her birth...luminous white shimmering gowns

Elane is aware of previous lives she has had, but knowing about them has not impacted her mission in this life, which is to write.

* * * * *

When Joan had a stroke, in her near-death experience she got to see her grandfather. He looked good, in his classic flannel shirt and baggy pants. He reassured her, "Don't be afraid. Everyone's here."

Transparent human-like beings pointed her to the left when she asked how to find her grandma, but she was not able to reach her before the experience ended.

"Jesus came to me and told me, 'You will never walk alone.'"

Her faith has been stronger since. She recognizes Jesus, but follows the Buddhist faith. "Buddha lived about the same time as Jesus."

* * * * *

Fatigue and malaise were replacing Rose's usual robust energy. When she sat to watch a Walt Disney World show, a well-dressed woman joined Rose. They chatted briefly. The woman then remarked, "I think you are going to die soon."

"I think you are going to die soon"

Before Rose could respond, the woman had slipped out of her seat and was down the aisle. The show had not even started.

Over the next few months, Rose fretted. Her fatigue worsened.

One night, Rose dreamt and worried about this. Her husband slept on the couch in her room and her sensitive dog slept on the bed with her. Suddenly, a stack of Walt Disney World boxes fell over for no reason. Amazingly, her husband and the dog were not aroused. She knew the house alarm system was working. Rose could not, for the life of her, explain what had caused the boxes to tumble.

Suddenly, there was a new noise. Boxes on the floor began to shuffle.

Boxes on the floor began to shuffle

Now Rose was trembling. She thought for sure there was a burglar. Her fear was overcome by an intense need to know. She got up.

The boxes were spread in a pattern that could not have resulted from their falling. But no one was around. Perplexed, she crawled back in bed. A voice spoke in her ear. But it was calm and reassuring. "You are not going to die. It was an evil force that said you were going to die." She was told to see me to begin healing. After a long process, she is much better.

* * * * *

Angelina, who was close to her sister, had a premonition with a stern warning that her brother-in-law Peter would die soon. Peter, who seemed very healthy, unexpectedly died three months later.

———

A high school girlfriend of Angelina's had broken up with a guy. The breakup had not gone well. Angelina had "hated" this guy since.

Six years later, he called her for a date. "I will hit him up for the max," Angelina thought, "a nice dinner AND a movie." On the way to dinner, she heard God say audibly, "You will marry him."

She was aghast! How could she ever marry him!

She did and has been happily married for 31 years.

* * * * *

Gertrude's boyfriend was incinerated in a car accident.

One night afterwards, Gertrude ran out through a hard rain and jumped in her car. She had a compelling urge to look into the rear view mirror. Her dead boyfriend smiled back at her.

Her dead boyfriend smiled back at her

"Drive carefully," he said. "Be safe."

Was her mind exhausted, playing tricks on her?

Time passed. Then once again she had to drive in the midst of a storm. Climbing in the car, she checked her mirror. There was his big smile. "Drive carefully. Be safe."

* * * * *

Dan's father died after his fifth heart attack at 45. Now Dan was not feeling well. He asked his wife to drive home.

He continued to sink. When home, Dan stretched out on the couch. "My wife said I turned white as a ghost. I could not move, could not speak and became unresponsive. I must not have been breathing because my wife beat on my chest."

Though comatose, he was able to observe all of this. He heard the Lord say, "It's your choice. You can go now." But he sensed the Lord was not ready for him yet. There were many reasons to stay.

Though comatose, he was able to observe... He heard the Lord say "It's your choice"

Dan recovered. His expanded ministry now includes addicts.

———

At church one night, Dan met Brother Johnson, who was speaking Sunday. God told Dan that Brother Johnson would be in the hospital Sunday. But Dan did not tell anyone.

Sunday morning, the minister called. Before he could get words out, Dan said, "It is Brother Johnson isn't it? He is in the hospital." He was.

———

Dan met Sierra who had been diagnosed with a pelvic tumor. Dan sensed she had been date-raped. He shared this with a friend who was counseling her. When the friend gently brought this up, Sierra proclaimed, "How did you know?" She had been date-raped by a friend of the family. Because of that, Sierra did not feel like she could tell anyone.

They had a "laying on of the hands" and prayer. Two weeks later, they could not find the tumor on CT scan.

* * * * *

When Rita was a graduate student, she left her body when sexually assaulted. Always intuitive, Rita dreamt of a death days before her grandfather's passing.

As a child, Rita had recurring dreams of a tornado sweeping through town. During the dream, she was restrained from going where she needed to go.

Later a tornado did strike Rita's town. She was in a downtown business when it struck. The storeowner kept her from going home while there was still time.

Most bothersome to Rita were vivid dreams of billowing smoke in the weeks leading up to 9/11. Two nights before that tragedy, she dreamt a specific image. It was a Middle Easterner in military clothing. When Osama Bin Laden's face appeared on TV following 9/11, she was shocked. It was the identical image.

...Vivid dreams of billowing smoke... leading up to 9/11

Frightened, she called her boyfriend, who lived two floors down in that apartment building. She would not leave his apartment for a long time.

(Many around the country were haunted by pre-9/11 premonitions.)

* * * * *

Sal had served in Afghanistan from the start. His life's goal had always been to spread as much positive karma as possible.

Roger was a war buddy whose close friendship was fostered by many close calls in fighting. Years later, he visited Sal after he developed pancreatic cancer. Roger knew he did not have much time. Sal was anxious to confirm the existence of "the other side." Roger made a deal where he promised he would connect in with Sal.

Since Roger died, "all kinds of crazy things have happened" at his house. Notable was the business card that kept levitating. His frightened wife kept slapping it down.

The business card kept levitating. His frightened wife kept slapping it down

* * * * *

James Medley at age two was hospitalized for pneumonia. His mother stayed close, almost never leaving his side. One morning, though, she was absent.

James rose from his body. Walls of his room were translucent and shimmering. A figure appeared. James eased back into his body and then quickly recovered. He has left his body three other times.

———

James' daughter was in a car accident while pregnant, resulting in birth two months early. The baby was born with a failing left kidney that had seven polyps.

James spent a half hour daily for two weeks in the nursery. One hand went over the crown chakra, the other over the base of the spine. The left arm takes negative energy while the right provides positive energy. James' left elbow was in an L shape to block negative energy from entering his body. He then shook it out as he left the hospital.

The plan was to operate on the bad kidney after two weeks. Before surgery, they repeated the scan. The left kidney had disappeared.

———

Martial artists can reach a spiritual level. James once lay on a bed of nails. Four concrete blocks were placed on his chest. They were smashed with a sledgehammer. You have to be in a spiritual place for this to work. If done "for show," it does not turn out well.

A bed of nails, four concrete blocks and a sledgehammer are not "for show"

* * * * *

Rosanne had developed severe heart failure. Her weight blossomed 50 pounds within days at the hospital.

Rosanne's skin was extraordinarily sensitive to touch. Despite her protests, hospital personnel were quite rough when turning her in bed. Phlebotomists seemed insensitive in handling her arm, compounded by her being such a tough "stick." As a registered nurse, Rosanne always sought to be careful with patients. This rough handling did not at all sit well!

She sank into a coma, but she could still hear. Doctors painted a hopeless picture to the family. Nurses traded off-hand comments that it was just a matter of time.

All of Rosanne's pain left. She was overcome with a sense of peace. Suddenly it hit her! This must mean she was dying. Immediately she "went into gear." She was not going down without a fight! Rosanne had too much to get done on earth. Most of all, she needed to be there for her dear grandchild. Rosanne clawed back. Finally, she awoke from her coma, which was unfortunate for hospital staff. She yelled at the doctors. She blistered the staff. How dare they talk that way about her while in a coma? Rosanne heard every hopeless word. Every negative, careless comment made her stew. She was scathing. "Never, ever speak that way around a comatose patient!"

"Never, ever speak that way around a comatose patient!"

* * * * *

Amelia was having difficulties with her husband Seth. She came home one night and found him smoking marijuana looking out the window. Intuitively, she knew he had been unfaithful.

She reacted in a predictably judgmental fashion. Where have you been? Do you realize what time it is? What's her name? What is keeping me from shoving you out the door? He was stone-faced.

Amelia was so hurt. She did not know what to do. Retreating to the bathroom, Amelia fervently told God she could not handle this herself.

Softly, a complete peace overcame her. Amelia went back out to her husband. Gently, she told him that she was going on up to bed. He could let her know if he needed anything. What amazed her is she was feeling, and speaking, without judgment.

Seth asked her to stay there with him. He rested his head on her chest. Both settled into a peaceful state.

* * * * *

Toni developed seizures after being abused as a child. She then became possessed. Toni spoke in several languages including Latin and Hebrew. When others prayed over Toni, she would have a seizure.

In a vivid dream, Toni saw what appeared to be her mother's face. It was not. It was a demon in disguise.

Looking the other direction she saw beautiful feet. She knew. They were Jesus' feet.

Her "possession" and Jesus' beautiful feet

Jesus' voice said to rebuke the demon. She did. Her mental state returned to normal. All seizures stopped. Six observers, including law enforcement, witnessed her "possession." Toni's husband, not a believer before, became "saved" following the demon's departure.

* * * * *

Ellen had a serene presence and glow as she began to tell her story. Ten years earlier, she had abdominal surgery. Afterwards, severe infection spread throughout her body. After entering Ellen's blood stream, it produced a life-threatening drop in blood pressure with organ failure. She lapsed into a coma. Her prognosis was so poor her mother was appointed power of attorney.

A custody battle ensued over her two children. Her drug-addicted ex-husband harassed Ellen's mother. This infuriated Ellen who heard all.

This infuriated Ellen who heard all. GOD: "Return to your children"

God told her, "Your work is not done. Return to your children."

She was determined to recover. Only *she* would take care of her children. Ellen healed completely.

Afterwards, she became intuitive. Ellen learned to follow God's lead. She heard when God directed her to move to Frankfort. It was a perfect move. Driving by a church, she said knowingly, "That's our church." Her life, the school and the church have all been great.

* * * * *

Wendy sometimes smells fresh blood or funeral flowers, a sign someone close to her will die within two months.

One night, in a vivid dream, she was in her sister's house. Her mother asked her to look after niece Samantha. Wendy was close to "Sam." Sam called Wendy to open a tight door. Wendy tugged, but could not get it to budge. When they turned around, smoke billowed from the ceiling. "Sam, stay by the door until it opens!" Soon the door opened.

The fire was happening real-time with her dream. While in her bed at home, Wendy's spirit was saving Sam.

The fire was real-time with her dream. Wendy's spirit saved Sam

* * * * *

Kit's husband was alcoholic. Repeatedly, he had been very abusive. When he passed out, Kit stood over him. She pointed a loaded gun.

You have heard the expression, "She was beside herself." Kit went out of body and stood beside herself. Her spiritual self talked her physical self out of the murder.

She has been happily married to her new husband for 16 years.

She pointed a loaded gun. She was literally beside herself

When Kit's second husband lost his job, they went through hard times. She questioned God. Kit needed to know she was worthy. She told God every time she saw a penny she would know her worthiness.

Afterwards, it seemed everywhere she looked she would find a penny. Her relatives complained, "Why had you not asked for quarters?"

Kit decided instead to ask for feathers. Now, she finds feathers everywhere. When she opened her car door, feathers flew out.

Her health suffering, Kit went from doctor to doctor seeking answers. All her tests turned out fine. "You are normal."

Before her visit with me, she found the tiniest feather. The feather gave her hope. It convinced her today's visit would lead to answers.

As she was on a single estrogen pill daily, I could predict all of the other symptoms Kit was likely experiencing: anxiety, panic, obsessive-compulsiveness, phobias, sleep disturbance, irritability, carbohydrate craving, low libido, breast pain, weight gain and migraines. As estrogen promotes autoimmune activity, I also predicted that she had bloating, brain fog, aches and pains in joints and muscles.

Kit smiled. God had been right. This is where she would find answers.

* * * * *

Kathy Rowland's calling is to teach talented students. Once when driving, she noticed a large white bird flying near her car. Jeremiah, a Hopi Indian spiritual adviser, interpreted the white bird as the angel Gabriel.

When driving near Louisville, the large white bird again appeared. Telepathically, the bird told her she must switch lanes. Kathy immediately responded. Had she stayed in that lane, a semi-truck would have crashed through her windshield.

A white bird said to switch lanes

Jeremiah has helped in other ways. When four, Kathy developed uncontrolled jerking – Tourette's syndrome, often caused by Lyme. Jeremiah determined something negative had happened in Kathy's life at that age, triggering these episodes. A Hopi ceremonial healing resolved her Tourette's episodes.

When Kathy was six, she nearly drowned. It was so traumatic she went out of body. Her soul could not be convinced to reenter her body. Jeremiah determined she had drowned in a ship in a previous life. That soul had to be retrieved. Once it joined Kathy's current soul, her spirit agreed to reenter her body.

* * * * *

Shirley Holbrock had serious challenges growing up. "At four years of age, I felt the presence of two eight-foot angelic people near my bed. I felt at peace and safe.

At church when I was little, the main platform collapsed, seriously injuring a woman's leg. I could see in the corner of the room a woman suspended in the air. That angel's presence allowed me to respond calmly to what was happening.

The angel's presence allowed me to respond calmly

Sixteen years ago I lost Sparkle, my one-eyed Belgian Malanois due to seizures. Recently in a nighttime vision while awake, I saw Sparkle as if in a movie. Just like when we would play hide and seek, Sparkle walked past me and pretended not to see me, then walked back by. I did not notice her having a bad eye.

When traveling back from Cincinnati, the Lord showed me an alternate way home. I ignored the advice to go my familiar way. My car was broadsided by a truck."

* * * * *

99

Sally's father was dying as Christmas approached. Suddenly, he began to see and talk to entities no one could see. Following these episodes, he became serene and upbeat. He was told by one entity that he would depart on two seven. Being December, the family assumed this would be December 27th. But that day came and went.

He would die on two seven

He did finally die – on February 7th.

At the graveyard, her cousin's daughter asked, "Mommy, what are all these people doing, some facing this way, others that way?"

"Who is that man and woman sitting on the bench (in army uniform and loop dress)?"

At home she asked, "Mommy, who are those two little children following you around?" She had miscarried twins.

* * * * *

Ann has had spiritual experiences and been out of body. Once Ann's rebellious niece Terry left the family very angry, shouting foul language as she walked out the door.

Years later, Ann had a compulsion to write Terry telling her how much she loved her. For a week, she strongly felt this urge. Suddenly, it stopped. Terry had committed suicide. Ann learned never to ignore her premonitions.

She then met Angie. Ann really liked Angie who was in a difficult financial bind. Because of her faith, Ann supported Angie. Often that is all that is needed. But some, like Angie, need more.

One night Ann awoke at three a.m. with an urge to contact Angie. Angie, though, did not have a phone. Ann climbed out of bed and was quickly on her way to Angie's house.

When she arrived, Angie thanked her. She was strongly contemplating suicide. Angie had been praying for Ann's comfort and reassurance.

* * * * *

Barbara had weight loss surgery and then became anemic. She visited doctor after doctor for help. None could find the answer. None would admit the original surgery might have been a problem.

Her condition deteriorated. Finally, Barbara was faced with surgery. She was told there was only a 25 percent chance of survival. She prayed fervently to God. Could he take her if she had no other work on earth? If she did have a mission to fulfill, "God let me live."

Before surgery, Barbara insisted the surgeon have blood cross-matched as a precaution. In fact, she insisted on hearing the order given over the phone.

During the surgery she left her body. From above, Barbara saw the surgeon start to sweat. Accidentally, he lacerated the spleen. She bled profusely. Then her heart stopped. As she watched in disbelief Barbara's thoughts raced. "Oh I've died! Is this what death is like?"

When she awoke in the recovery room, Barbara was ecstatic. "I'm alive!" The nurses looked around startled. Barbara shouted to the rooftops, "I'm really alive!"

She watched in disbelief "I've died! Is this what death is like?"

* * * * *

Amy was in a head-on car collision. The car's mangled metal wrapped around her. Smoke billowed from the front.

Amy felt a wave of fear. Thoughts bombarded her. Would the car burst into flames? Would it consume her? Would she die?

Then a voice spoke clearly. "You are not going to die."

Shortly, Mark, who was driving the pickup behind her, came to Amy's car door. "Can I help you?" With much effort, Mark's strong frame tugged at her body. Slowly, Amy slid through the crumpled window.

* * * * *

Laura was having an imaging study due to a suspected compression fracture in her back. The pain was incredibly intense. They kept saying, "Hang in there," but she replied, "No, I am not able."

Then Laura coded. While they wheeled in an emergency cart, she went into a very wonderful state of mind. Suddenly, she realized this incredible feeling meant she was dying! "No!" she told herself. "I've got to take care of my children. I must go back!" Immediately, she returned to consciousness.

———

Laura was driving safely at 50 mph when a drunken truck driver going 95 mph approached from the other direction. In the second before head on impact, something seemingly unfathomable happened. Both Laura and her son saw it. There was an angel on both sides of the car. Everything went into slow motion. The car slowly slid into the median.

My son and I saw an angel on both sides of the car guide it to safety

The "Jaws of Death" was needed to get Laura and her son out of the car, but they both emerged alive and with all parts.

* * * * *

As a practitioner in New Mexico, Daniel focused on helping troubled patients. Other healers had heard glowing reports of his success.

A young girl, Sonora, had sudden changes in behavior. Her voice would become very deep. She would spew angry, vitriolic words. Sonora said two demons were entering her body at those times.

Two demons were entering her body

Sonora's mother brought her to Daniel. During the visit, Sonora saw the demons enter her body. Her voice became very deep and angry.

"God is very bad! You are always expected to do what God wants. Ignore God, do what *you* want to do!"

This was clearly not a six-year-old voice. Daniel was shocked, but kept his composure. From somewhere words came to him. "When God gives you presents, he does not give you a gun. That would be wrong."

"When you buy school clothes, you don't get a miner's uniform. That would be inappropriate. God sees that you get what you need, but only the right types of things, not ones that are strange or harmful."

After more angry words, Sonora's demeanor suddenly shifted. She was back to the little girl. Daniel gave a fervent prayer for her healing.

* * * * *

Dawna Plummer experiences a knowing of others and has visions in her dreams. She got a call from a friend to join a group gathering to pray for someone who was occupied by demons. At the house, she saw a 10-foot angel dressed like a warrior with a sword. She made a comment to him and he replied, "It is a fashion statement."

"When deep in prayer I saw myself following Jesus on a path. He was dressed in a robe and sandals. I could not see his face. He began walking away, then turned and said, 'Tell them I am coming soon.'"

Jesus: "Tell them I'm coming soon"

Another time when praying, Dawna found herself in an old town from the time of Jesus. As she walked with Jesus, she could smell the dirt, the horses and other scents.

When praying in a group, she noticed something on her nose. When they were through with the prayers, others commented about the gold dust on her nose.

* * * * *

At 27 years old, Mary Moraja experienced cardiac tamponade – accumulation of blood in the sac around the heart strangling it. She found herself in the corner watching as doctors were working on some woman down below. Then she realized – that was her!

Mary was being drawn to the light. She felt incredible peace unlike any other she has ever experienced. She sensed other beings including her deceased brother and grandparents.

She had a choice to go on or to come back. She started to go on when she remembered her three-year-old child and her terrible husband. She decided she had to come back. After blood was drawn out of her heart, she had a full recovery.

She sensed her dead grandparents

She has no longer feared death, a fact that has likely been instrumental in thriving survival from subsequent cancer.

* * * * *

Sherry's house was custom made, with the baby's room right next to hers. The door was kept ajar. Every sound could be monitored.

Sherry's husband had left town. Her baby required feeding through the night due to fussiness. Sherry was sleeping soundly.

In the middle of the night, a light suddenly flipped on in the baby's room. Then a voice. "She is in there."

Sherry froze in her bed.

A seven-foot white entity glided into her room. Was it an angel? She could not tell. The hair was long and gray.

A seven-foot white entity glided into her room and put its hand on her forehead

The entity put its hand on her forehead. "Spirit of Mercy" came from its lips. Then it floated away.

Sherry continued in a frozen state, unable to get out of bed. There was not a sound from the next room. What happened to her baby? It always woke up fussy. But not a sound.

How could she convince herself this whole episode was real? She decided to keep her eyes wide open all night.

Finally at nine a.m., the spell wore off. She rushed out of bed terrified. Had something happened to the baby? Was it still there?

She found her baby sleeping peacefully. Why had her baby not fussed? Ever since her baby has slept well.

* * * * *

Dale was three years old sitting behind a couch cross-legged.

Suddenly, from his right upper field of vision, came what seemed like thousands of faces, one after the other. Speeding toward him, each face flitted through his mind and exited to his upper left, absorbing in a brief instant everything he knew and had experienced in his brief life.

From his upper right came what seemed like thousands of faces

Immediately, Dale experienced a "knowing" that these were spiritual entities. Every question that came to mind was instantly answered telepathically - whole thoughts were exchanged without any use of words. He asked if his mind would be controlled. "No, you have free will. During your life, you will encounter situations in which you must decide on the right thing to do. We will be especially interested in your decisions when you are not sure what is best."

Dale asked why they were doing this. They replied it was part of a great experiment. They reassured him they would always be with him. They ended the episode saying, "Do not fear, we hold no harm for you, only good will. We love you. You, little spirit, are one of us, but you may not speak with us, or understand why you have this purpose, until your life has been lived out and you join us."

"You, little spirit, are one of us"

Dale says this early childhood experience has profoundly influenced his long life. He has always felt compelled to seek fuller understanding of a unity of spirituality, nature and human purpose. He now understands "purpose" to mean helping others and attaining knowledge.

* * * * *

Carolyn had a younger brother, Todd, who was very short. She thought of him as a leprechaun. Todd had died at an early age.

Her granddaughter Joy had a miscarriage at eight months, but had named the baby Ava. Shortly afterwards, she saw a vision of her "leprechaun" brother Todd with Ava, now appearing two years old. Ava was riding on Todd's shoulders. She kept asking Todd to come to her, but teasingly he kept dancing around just out of reach. Then they disappeared.

———

Carolyn's prayer group forms a circle. One day from the opposite side of the circle, Carolyn saw Jesus approach her. His arms were open to embrace her. She rose to embrace him.

Suddenly, a dog ran from behind Jesus. It was her dearly beloved Bruno, who had recently died. When Carolyn embraced Jesus, he and Bruno both vaporized.

Her dead dog ran from behind Jesus

* * * * *

A recurring lung infection flared, and June's fever surged. She struggled to catch her breath. June was frightened. She did what she always did in these frantic situations – she prayed.

Then he came. Jesus sat in the corner of the room.

She asked him to come next to her bed so she could rest her hand on his knee. June could feel the tassel from his robe.

She felt the tassel from Jesus' robe

Later that night, a severe pain suddenly shot through her right pelvis. Jesus reached his hand into her body, pulled out that painful area and turned it in his hand. It developed a beautiful emerald hue. Then, he placed it back. Her pain immediately dissolved. Jesus told her that while her lung problems were life threatening, she would not die from them.

Jesus' hand reached into her body

* * * * *

Mack McAdams when 20 was run over by a female emergency medical technician (EMT) as she was headed to work. He went through a tunnel as if he was passing through a birth canal being reborn, headed toward the light. He felt exquisitely peaceful, beyond anything he could describe.

When the EMT started CPR, Mack came back from the tunnel, hovering on the wires near a light pole watching down below. When he realized how devastating his death would be to his mother, he knew he had to come back.

Since then, according to a family member, he has been very giving. "He would give you anything!" He no longer fears death and has become intuitive.

_____

He once developed pneumonia and his lungs filled with fluid. Mack heard the doctor say that he only had 48 hours to live.

This time in his near-death state, Mack was in a valley with everything still. It was the "Valley of Death," between being and non-being. It was a red-orange color. He sensed both God and death.

It was the "Valley of Death"

Mack asked if he could see his daughter before he died. He knew if he passed 48 hours he would make it. As it took her more than 48 hours to reach him, he knew he would live.

_____

Mack was working security when a woman with a little girl passed him in the hall. "Are you thinking of having another child?" As she turned toward him, he added, "You will have a boy."

She was on the way to the doctor to see if she was pregnant and was incredulous that he knew. Ultrasound later confirmed a boy.

* * * * *

Katie Goldey had a vivid dream. "I was lying in a field at dawn." She heard a plane. It was flying too low. She worriedly told her companion, "That plane is flying way too low. It is going to crash!"

Within hours of that dream and less than 10 miles away, a regional plane crashed at the Lexington airport, killing all aboard but the pilot. The plane, taking off on a closed shortened runway, crashed into trees before it could gain sufficient altitude.

Her vivid dream premonition of the Lexington plane disaster

One day when talking to her grandmother, Katie had the vision of scissors gorily puncturing her grandmother's chest. The next day, her grandmother had a heart attack.

At the King's Island amusement park, Katie normally loved riding the roller coasters. But this particular day she had recurring images of wheels and blood so she did not ride one all day. That day it turned out that the son of her dad's friend from high school fell off a float and was run over by the float's wheels.

* * * * *

Jennifer made some highly regrettable decisions. Her mood sank until she was suicidal. With a Bible on one side and a gun on the other, Jennifer sat contemplating. She put the gun to her head.

"Don't shoot."

Startled, Jennifer jumped up. She searched the room, then the hallway. The house was empty. No one was around. She sat down. Again, Jennifer pointed the pistol.

"Don't shoot, daughter!"

"Don't shoot, daughter!"

Now she knew. This was her heavenly father. Jennifer put the gun down. She fell to her knees praying.

* * * * *

Peggy was doing a self-exam when she found a breast lump. Unsure of its importance, she decided to monitor it for a week. That night, during a vivid dream, she was suddenly awakened by a gravelly voice saying, "You have breast cancer."

Her physician evaluated the lump. She felt it to be benign. Subsequently, it appeared to disappear altogether. But weeks later, the lump returned. It was prior to her next menstrual cycle, a time when non-cancerous lumps sometimes enlarge.

Peggy, however, had another frightening dream. She was woken by a sinister voice that sent chills down her spine. It scowled, "You have one week to live!"

A sinister voice scowled: "You have one week to live!"

Peggy was very confused and scared. Her sleep became restless. She would take long naps during the day. During a "more real than life" dream, she saw clouds parting. A warm, powerful presence descended upon her. A beautiful voice said reassuringly, "All is well." Peggy had a "knowing" that it was a true and divine message. Her worries completely melted away.

The physician, as a precaution, did a biopsy. As it was suspicious, the surgeon removed it. There was no evidence whatsoever of cancer.

* * * * *

Ron had inoperable lung cancer. A year earlier, he arose at four a.m. to get to work. He did not feel well, but pushed himself to get there. As had been true for years, he was first to arrive at work. When his friend Ken arrived, Ron suddenly collapsed.

At the hospital, Ron was given a morphine shot. His heart stopped. Ron was in a tunnel. At the very end was a light. A woman stood in the light with an outstretched hand, waiting.

Ron did not recognize her. With much effort, he made it through. Immediately, there was a beautiful feeling. Ron sensed complete love. The incredible beauty surrounding him was overwhelming.

There before him was the Pearly Gate. Jesus greeted him.

There before him was the Pearly Gate

Soon, Jesus shared it was not his time. Ron would have to go back. Swoosh! He felt himself being sucked back in to his body.

Ron agreed: this realm was more "real" than earthly experience. When visiting the home of his wife's family, Ron was shown a picture of his wife's best friend. He recognized her immediately. It was the woman who had welcomed him at the tunnel's end.

At his office visit, Ron was radiant. Though he recognized that his friends and family wanted to hold on to him, Ron was now ready to die.

* * * * *

Shirley Witt, a sweet, sharp elder, shared that when she was 18, God told her that when the end came, Jesus was going to be taking her up with the others in his group.

When she was shown a house to consider for purchase, it had a room with yellow paint in it so she did not want the house. God told her that was OK, to buy it anyway. She and her husband did, and they lived in it for many wonderful decades since.

She needed to get a new roof and had contacted seven contractors, but none of them were "worth a hill of beans." She was worried and didn't know what to do. She prayed for help.

When driving down the street, she felt a "stovepipe" of spirit envelop her. When she hit a certain point on a street, it disappeared. She was next to a house that was getting a roof. There was one parking spot out front, just big enough for her car. She got out to speak with the foreman. They did a good job repairing her roof.

She had let her yard go for three years. One day in reflecting how drab it looked, she could not stop apologizing to Jesus. She apologized at least four times. She worked hard that fall and the next spring. The next year's flowers bloomed brightly and the yard was beautiful. She said to Jesus, "Aren't you pleased now at how the yard looks?" Immediately, an image of Jesus flashed onto a nearby tree; then instantly it disappeared.

Jesus' image flashed on a tree

* * * * *

"I died when 19 years old, likely due to a brain aneurysm. On a beautiful Sunday afternoon, I had gone to my boyfriend's house. While preparing lunch together in his kitchen I felt an explosion in my head with the most excruciating pain ever. The man I would marry says I fell backwards, my head bouncing against the tile floor. My body went into convulsions, and then I died. My heart stopped. Trained in CPR, he pumped my chest, yelled for his roommate and urgently called my name.

All I knew at the time was I went somewhere else. All was calm and peaceful. Language makes describing a near-death experience difficult because we do not have words that encompass the feel/texture of souls, nor even what God is like. Calling the presence of God a force, or a light, does not do justice to what it actually is, but we are limited by a vocabulary created in the physical world in which we live. I was met by 'people' or, in other words, other souls with a soft milky feel to them.

I was met by…souls with a soft milky feel to them

I realized many things at once about this non-physical plane of existence. I was well aware that there were distant souls that were more prickly and scary. But those were not the ones surrounding me. I understood that the physical concept I had of pure heaven and pure hell may not have been accurate since there are different states of souls. Still, I was certainly glad I was not in the state of the prickly/scary, 'tortured' souls. An outside force was not torturing those souls. They are tortured souls because they already were tortured souls when they died. I understood that the afterlife cannot get crowded with souls the way our planet could get crowded with people. I understood in an instant the infinite nature of this other existence. We simply do not have words nor are we able to adequately grasp the non-physical nature of the after-life.

The light was there to embrace me, but I was being given a choice. I could return to my body. I did not want to. I wanted to stay with the light. I was allowed to be aware of the other plane of existence - the physical one - in which the man I loved, and who loved me so, was calling my name, insistently, despairingly. I felt torn. But I chose to 'come back' only because love was calling me back.

I returned to an ocean of pain. I could not move or speak, but I was told my heart was again beating and I was moaning. I do not 'believe' in souls and God. I unshakably KNOW we have souls and that we are a part of God."

-Jeanie Wolfson, Author of *It's Not Mental*

* * * * *

"We were lying in bed the night before my husband, Todd, would embark on his 10-day trip to Rwanda, Africa, a 24-hour flight by himself. This would be only his second time out of the country and by far the longest trip ever away from our three young children and me. The flight would be ending in Kigali, Africa where a Congolese friend would be meeting my husband. We talked about the trip, our fears and anxieties and how we would be in touch with each other given the six-hour time difference. Soon after that I fell asleep quickly as I usually do, but in the middle of the night I kept getting stirred awake by a voice I have come to know well over the years.

God gives me impressions, usually at night, through the Holy Spirit. The words and visions I receive I always test to the character of God, which is only and always good. My discernment and obedience to God's voice has given my husband great confidence in my gifting and hearing from The Lord. I was awoken several times that night with this word: FEARLESS. Knowing that when God is persistent it is always for a good reason, I became more alert to his nudging me and I questioned silently to God, 'What does this mean?' I felt again this impression from The Lord: 'I call Todd fearless, not in an unfearing way toward me (God), but fearless that he should be courageous, and not have fear because I, The Father, am with him.'

I finally rolled over and asked Todd if he was awake; he groggingly replied yes. I told him what The Lord had said to me exactly, and then I rolled back over and went to sleep, completely at peace.

That morning was hectic as usual and we all parted ways to school and to work. Later that night when Todd came home and began preparing for the flight, I asked if he remembered me telling him anything the night before. He replied yes, that he had been lying there in that moment consumed by anxiety and fear about his long flight and the many unknowns of the trip itself. After I shared that God was calling him fearless, he was relieved and instantly at peace. He had gone into work that morning and shared what happened that night with his colleagues. Because of that, he knew he could step into his journey to Rwanda FEARLESS, with complete confidence in God's peace and God's presence with him!

"GOD was calling him fearless"

Just a simple reminder that we should all be fearless as God's children! 'We know that all things work together for the good of those who love God-those whom He has called according to His plan,' Romans 8:28."

-Jenny Clayton, LMT

* * * * *

"I remember meeting a lady at a church where my husband and I were ministering. On introduction, the lady said, 'Oh I know Annette, I met her in one of my dreams.' Odd. But true and so cool.

About 10 years ago at The Rock Worship Center in Somerset, Kentucky, I was teaching Sunday school for the six to eight-year-olds. I requested they introduce themselves to the new young boy. This six-year-old boy says to Kayla, who was 12, 'You do not need to tell me who you are, because I met you in a field of flowers and your name is Kayla!' I knew he was telling the truth because of the experience I had already had with someone meeting me in a dream.

A few years back, I was at dinner with two friends. On the way home, we were involved in an auto accident in Cincinnati. As our car was spinning out of control, suddenly my spirit left my physical body and was hovering outside the car on the right front side of the windshield. Through the windshield, I watched the three bodies react to the impact in slow motion, bouncing around. I was at perfect peace. When the auto stopped, my spirit went back into my body.

A year ago, I was at the local post office. As I stepped up to the window, I told the lady helping me, 'I know that you think that I am here because physically I am, but spiritually I am not. I am actually at the Union Terminal in Cincinnati speaking with the young lady at the informational desk.' The lady at the post office said to my surprise, 'I am so glad that you told me.' She had recently had such an encounter herself and thought that she was going bonkers.

"It was as if my passenger, me and my car moved (from) one dimension to another..."

About 20 years ago, I was able to take my car through two other cars. I was drag racing and there was no other way to win except to go through the two cars blocking my car. It was as if my passenger, me and my CAR moved through one dimension to another dimension. How? I do not know, other than in my mind I just knew I could, so I did. My passenger was in shock. The odd thing about it, many years later I was at a meeting and shared the experience with a group of ladies, and as I was explaining the experience a lady named Bonnie said to me that she was driving down the expressway in Northern Kentucky when a car appeared to have gone though the car that she and her daughter were in. When I questioned her further, I do believe that she was one of the cars that were involved, because it happened on the same expressway at the same location."

-Annette West

* * * * *

Deborah was unable to heal serious eye problems. Rosemary, the healer, did a "scan" of Deborah's body noting several organs were holding wounds from memories that would lead to illness. She wanted to heal those before dealing with the eye problems. As Rosemary worked, Deborah could feel the work deep inside her body. Rosemary helped Deborah recall a preverbal memory that explained her relationship to her parents as a young child and subsequent challenges.

As Rosemary moved to Deborah's heart, all at once Deborah felt release from her heart, tension eased and a billowing dirty yellow cloud poured out of her chest, swirling above her. Leaving the room to protect herself from the toxic energy, Rosemary instructed Deborah to urge the cloud out. "Envision replacing it with a color flowing around your heart." Deborah envisioned a turquoise color.

A billowing dirty yellow cloud poured out of her chest

She was filled with understanding about the incident that closed her heart, allowing negativity to reside there – an incident she often remembered, but only then understood its profound significance. She was 17. It was her last conversation with her beloved grandfather. Before dying, he apologized for not being able to stay and protect her from a destructive family member. Once she understood, Deborah released her sense of insecurity and abandonment, replacing it with contentment and gratitude for such a talented, dedicated servant.

––––––

Deborah's father Art was an intelligent, complicated, difficult man. His volatile temper created an emotionally unsafe home. Her sisters were in constant conflict with him. Her older sister severed all contact with him when she had her own family. Deborah survived by being as small and quiet as possible. Even so her sisters accused her of being "Daddy's favorite."

As she matured, Deborah could see that her father sought to fill a void. In time she understood that although a proclaimed agnostic, Art searched for spiritual fulfillment. As Deborah moved on her own spiritual path, her father became ever more curious. That ended when Art had a heart attack. Deborah heard from others that when EMTs started his heart after he had "died," he was angry at being pulled out of that dark tunnel before he reached the light. He had never felt so completely accepted and loved without judgment. His final transition came two weeks later.

Over the following decades, Deborah frequently thought of her father's experience. She grieved that she was not there to witness his story. She wondered what he was experiencing on the other side. She finally got her wish 32 years after his transition.

Deborah awoke suddenly at three a.m. Afraid she would not fall back to sleep, she went to the living room to meditate. The moonlit scenery streamed through the windows. Finally, her eyes closed to meditate. Instead, behind her closed eyes, a universe of pastel colors swirled. As she watched, flat concentric squares appeared, alternating between being perfectly clear and being slightly richer than the pastel background. Suddenly, the squares expanded out away from her like an accordion. Behind the furthest tiny square, a bright white light appeared that grew ever larger behind the squares. Somehow, she knew her father was there.

"Dad, is that you?" "Yes," he answered. "What is this about?" Deborah asked. "You can come now if you want to," he replied. Deborah was shocked. Was he saying she could die and join him right then? After years of depression, she was finally emotionally healthy. She did not want to die. She opened her eyes, but quickly realized she might have misunderstood. But when she closed them again, she could not reconnect with that vision.

Her dead dad: "You can come now"

For weeks she sought an explanation. Deborah asked everyone she could trust what they thought he had meant. One night a friend replied, "Why don't you ask him yourself? He is right here in the room." Startled, through her friend who did not know her family history, she learned her father meant Deborah was close to another state of consciousness. She was standing in her own way. He gave instructions on how to proceed. She asked her dad if he knew what had happened to her older sister who died before reconnecting with her banished father. For all of her 48 years, her sister had been angry and divisive. Deborah hoped she had found peace. Her father explained that just before she had the stroke she had "surrendered." During the eight weeks in a coma and six days she survived after removal of life support, she had worked with her angels, guides and teachers to prepare for an easier transition to the other side. She was teaching other new arrivals what she had learned. Deborah was so relieved. Then her father disappeared.

She had worked with her angels, guides and teachers for transition

Deborah was to hear from her father two more times when she was alone and could see him. One time he shared he had chosen to die when he had so other members of his family could move on with their lives without being in constant conflict with, and about, him. He told her he had always been with her and her children whom he never knew; sometimes he assisted in troubled times. When he last appeared, he was smiling. "I want you to know I am proud of you and how you have evolved. I came into our shared lifetime to point you to the work you have been preparing to do for the world. I know you will do it and do it well." Then he was gone.

For Deborah, her father's visits brought closure. It relieved her grief from not being present in his last days. She was comforted knowing for sure that his soul survived. Both he and her sister were at peace on the other side. She was overwhelmed with emotion about his presence in her and her family's lives. Someday their souls will meet again and she will share that fuller experience she longs for.

* * * * *

"While living in Southwest England at age 22, I traveled to Oxford to stay with a friend. During the drive up to her home, I began to ache and, by the time I realized, I was suddenly very ill. I was closer to her home than mine so I kept heading her way. Opening the door, she took one look at me and sent me straight to bed. I remember feeling very hot, I must have drunk a gallon of water and my temperature read a little over 104F. I had a very sharp pain in my abdominal area and was shaking uncontrollably.

Perhaps I should have gone straight to the hospital, but I was young and in a foreign land and my host offered a free alternative. My friend's father happened to be the bishop of the district we were in and knew of a healer who had been a member of one of the churches under his care. I remember thinking, my friend has lost her mind when she suggested calling Mary the healer to her home to help me, but I was in so much pain and agony that I agreed.

When Mary arrived about an hour later, I was lying on a pallet on the floor. She never spoke to me; she just kneeled beside me and said a prayer out loud. Then she placed her hands a few inches above my clothing and began to slowly move them up and down over my body. I remember her eyes were closed. I felt complete shock when she stopped her hands over the exact area where most of my pain was centered: how did she know? She spoke another prayer and in that moment, I felt comfort and peace and my shaking ceased.

"I felt complete shock when she stopped her hands over the exact area...of my pain"

Mary looked at me and began to tell me things about my recent risky behavior and actions that were hurting my soul. How did this stranger know?! I had been partying too much, hanging out with the wrong characters, gotten away from my spiritual center. She offered advice on getting back to good spiritual health and I took it seriously. Mary left the room and as I heard the front door close, I felt the energy dissipate and my condition relapsed somewhat, but I continued to focus on what she told me. By the next day I was well. I have entered my late thirties and I often still call up that event in my mind as a reminder of the power of prayer and spiritual healing. I feel a deep connection to my inner voice and trust my instincts and intuition, believing that we all have a sixth sense, and the power to heal and connect to a higher power."

-Erin Sullivan

* * * * *

Sienna went to the hospital with a severe gallbladder infection. A stone had lodged in her bile duct, blocking healing. Surgery would be necessary. Sienna was apprehensive. As she lay on the gurney waiting for the anesthesiologist, Selena drifted into a different realm.

Incredibly, she recognized that she had entered heaven.

Sienna walked on vividly green grass. She waded through a nearby stream. Every direction was visible at once. Selena could see Jesus; he was talking with someone. She then entered a bubble guided by an angel and was given a tour of hell. There she saw unhappy people in prison and other very tragic things.

She entered a bubble guided by an angel, and was given a tour of hell

Back in heaven, she saw 12 entrances. When asked if she thought this was one for each religion, Sienna thought they might be entrances for different personalities. She was able to open her eyes and exit the scenario, then close them and reenter it.

* * * * *

In for his first visit, Joseph had lived a full life. Now old, he had been diagnosed with advanced pancreatic cancer. When I shared it was important he be at peace, I told of my many patients with near-death experiences. He thanked me for saying this. "It is important that you share this with others and write a book."

"It is important that you share this with others and write a book"

Joseph had an amazing thing happen. One night he had a very vivid dream. In the dream, his friend Thomas was on the fifth floor of Central Baptist hospital with a heart attack. Three friends were attending him. Subsequently, in the dream Thomas died.

Joseph woke with an incredible sense of peace. It was beyond anything he had ever experienced. It was so special that he did not want to leave bed lest he lose that feeling. Gradually, the feeling subsided. Joseph went down for breakfast.

His wife said there had been a phone call. His friend Thomas had been admitted to the hospital. He was on the fifth floor of Central Baptist. Thomas had suffered a serious heart attack.

An incredibly striking premonition

When he went to visit Thomas, the three friends he had seen in his dream were there with him. Joseph shared the story with Thomas' wife, Elise. Except he left out the part that Thomas died.

Days later, Thomas did die. Joseph then apologized to Elise. He did not know how to tell her Thomas had died in his dream.

* * * * *

When brother-in-law Rene came by the house, Lori was mowing the yard. He seemed to speak in slow motion. She thought it was her hormones. Rene asked Lori to ride with him on an errand.

Lori's hands froze to the lawnmower. She could not pull them loose. She told Rene to go ahead, while she mowed.

Lori's hands froze to the lawnmower. She could not pull them lose

Soon afterwards, Lori had a sinking feeling. Soon, sirens wailed in the distance. Rene's accident was fatal.

———

At Christmas, Lori was peacefully resting when words came. She wrote them down. They were from Rene. It was a message for his wife.

Afraid this would upset her, Lori placed the words in her sister Kate's Bible. She told her to read them later.

Kate called to tell her she had been praying for answers about Rene. These words wondrously provided them. Kate was extremely grateful.

* * * * *

Danielle was divorced from her husband. She now lived alone.

She would frequently notice a shadow in her house. It was that of a tall military figure. He wore a long trench coat and large military hat.

Behind her house was an old cemetery. Once Danielle saw the shadow rise from a cemetery grave and enter her house. In fact, when she went in the front door, the shadow came in through the back door. At night after she went to bed, he would stand in the doorway between the bedroom and bathroom.

One night when asleep, Danielle felt a tugging at her nightgown. The shadow was warning her. Danielle's ex-husband had just parked his car in front of her house.

The shadow was warning her

The shadow was her protector. With the shadow around, she was always comforted. It was difficult, years later, to move away. She missed his company.

* * * * *

"Forty-one years ago my pregnancy with my second child was very stormy. Three months after his birth I was still bleeding; therefore, I underwent a fairly routine D & C. I was brought back to my room and with the bed rails up, happily and peacefully continued sleeping off the anesthesia.

After a while I noted that it would be a really good idea if I could empty my bladder. Being young and with no nursing experience at the time, I thought I could probably crawl over the rails, but decided I really wasn't up to the task! I rang the call bell and eventually a nurse came to my bedside at which time I explained that I really needed to use the bathroom. She decided that she should check me first; in doing so she discovered she was already standing in a pool of blood. She panicked and ran out of the room shouting at me not to move. I could hear my room number being announced on the intercom along with my doctor's name.

It seemed like seconds that an entire team of nurses had surrounded my bed hovering over me along with my doctor. As he applied pressure to my lower abdomen trying to see if there were any clots, my spirit immediately went right up. It is amazing to me the clarity of my thoughts as my spirit was looking down at the tops of everyone's heads and my lifeless body. I clearly remember thinking about my new baby and my precious four-year-old along with the difficulty my leaving two small boys might bring to my husband. However, I instantly consoled myself with the thought that my husband's sister only lived a few houses down from us and that it would be okay. I distinctly remember a very peaceful feeling and knew I was smiling!

The cubicle in the four-bed ward did not allow privacy except for pulled curtains. However, at the time it seemed as if my medical team and I were the only people in the room. Everything seemed very dark around us with ample bright light within my little cubicle. It seemed as if my spirit was almost against the wall as it had gone straight up with my toes still touching my shoulders. As I received an injection in each arm my spirit slid right back down and positioned itself at the ends of my fingers and to the tips of my toes. I describe it as if a person had a fine laser and tried to shine it in the center of a spot on the wall; you might move it up or down or round and round until you find the exact center of the spot. My spirit seemed to be more like a shadow as I hesitate to say dark.

I can recall that experience at this moment as if it happened a moment ago. I have never lost the clarity of the event, even though there are other events in my life that I have lost details due to time.

"...My spirit... positioned itself at the ends of my fingers and to the tips of my toes"

What did I learn from this experience? My first experience with death was when my grandfather died. In my 11-year-old brain, I could not reconcile myself with the fact that he was no longer alive. He died right after I was supposed to spend a week with him, and I chose a cousin's house instead. I felt maybe his death was my fault, I felt guilty, I had no understanding, it seemed unfair and where in the world did he go?

Then a year after my husband and I were married, my husband's father died. He, like my grandfather, was one of the sweetest, humblest men I had ever met. He was a missionary minister and was disabled due to losing a leg in the mines, and after he was able to walk with a prosthesis, he was hit by a drunk driver and the other leg was mangled. Now how could he possibly deserve to die?

Those two experiences were very haunting to me and I had a very difficult time thinking death could be a part of life. It seemed as a punishment that happened to wonderful people.

The bleeding vessel that caused my event was repaired, I was given a couple pints of blood and I was roomed with a young mother who I had never met. We discovered that she had gone to high school with my husband and lived near our home. Somehow we got on the subject of what happens when we die. She was a member of The Church of Jesus Christ of Latter Day Saints. I studied their beliefs for over a year, and my questions about death and many more questions I had for years were answered. Our life has been built around our beliefs, which bring me much comfort and satisfaction. I believe I was being prepared for the future, as we later had nine deaths in our family in two years. I also lost someone that seemed to take a little of me with them and left me broken for quite some time.

She knew about my experience and had some of her own. I long for her every day, but due to my experience, I know that I will live on in the next life and be with her again."

-Claudean Oakley

* * * * *

"From the age of five I had a special friend who was my neighbor, school principal, Sunday School teacher, surrogate grandmother and later on my professional mentor, all rolled into one little woman.

Her name was Mable Doggett. She was 15 years older than my mother, a bit Victorian, and had a younger sister the age of my mother, named Margaret, who was more like a big sister to me. They were both single.

Their home was like a second home to me, for they both doted on me, and each claimed me as 'the daughter we never had.' How my heart would swell when they took me on trips and introduced me as 'our girl' with great pride and love in their voices. They were very special, and I loved them both very much.

My mother often remarked how thankful she was that they were in my life, helping her raise me properly, for they, especially Mable, were role models. She was like a Pied Piper, devoting her entire life to the care and education of children, and was revered in our city, Kingsport, TN.

As I matured, worked, married, moved away and had children of my own, I treasured and nurtured our relationship, giving Mable special attention as she aged, so that she would never feel forgotten. She had other protégés, but only a few remembered what this special lady had done for them.

Finally, in the early 70s, Mable had to go into a nursing home. She was suffering dementia, and Margaret was no longer able to care for her. On my visits home, I would always go to see her and even in her fog she would know me. I relate all this just to establish how close we were, and how we loved each other.

On Nov. 1, 1974, at Ft. Sill, Oklahoma I was awakened by a vivid dream. Something told me to look at the clock. It was 1:10 a.m. In the dream, a passenger train was going through our front yard, and I was standing on our screened-in porch. Mable was holding the bar at one of the car doors and leaning out of it, calling loudly to me, 'GOODBYE, ANNE! GOODBYE, ANNE!' as she waved with her free hand, the train moving on and gradually her voice fading away as I awoke.

I knew somehow that Mable had died. I woke my husband, but could not bring myself to say that Mable was dead. I could only say, 'Mable is...not...going to make it.' He and I both went back to sleep.

At 8:00 our phone rang. I answered, and it was my mother. As soon as I heard her voice I knew what she was about to tell me, but I didn't give her a chance. I just asked, 'What time did she die?' Mother answered, 'At 2:10 this morning,' which, with the time zone difference, was the exact moment I awoke from the dream and looked at my clock.

I flew back to Tennessee for the funeral, and of course sought out Margaret. I told her about my dream.

Margaret's eyes grew large and her face incredulously serious, and she said to me, while holding up four fingers, 'You are the fourth person to tell me of this!'

"Margaret's eyes grew large and her face incredulously serious..."

We just stared at each other for a moment, then Margaret told me the names of the three others, all of whom I knew about having been protégés of Mable's, even though I had never met them. We all lived in different time zones, but all had the same dream at the very same time! I wish I had written down their names, but I didn't think to do that, and now Margaret is gone, too, so I can't ask her.

So, why would our Creator allow that dream to happen that way? I don't know, but I sometimes wonder if He allowed it just to let me have the comfort of feeling so very loved by Mable....that I really was special to her, and that what had happened was very, very real. I certainly needed affirmation of being loved at that time.

There was another time when I heard Mable's voice in 1978, but that will be in another book."

-Anne Wood

My Office and Miraculous Rescues

Surrounded by God's Presence, I have been greatly blessed by the wonderful people at work. Laughter echoes down the halls daily. Our blessings are now apparent.

While visiting Germany with her children, another family joined them. Anita's mind suddenly bolted to the corner of the room. For 10 minutes she watched herself below, talking to the other mother. "It was the oddest feeling."

Anita's first out of body experience occurred after delivery of a child. She did not know why this happened or what to make of it. After a third experience, Anita decided these needed to stop. Following osteopathic manipulation, they have ceased.

* * * * *

Christy Pellegrino's beloved brother Kelly had advanced multiple myeloma. She had a vivid dream where she saw his silhouette in a brown chair under the care of hospice. Three months later, he was admitted to hospice. When she visited, there he was, his silhouette in that brown chair just the way she had visualized it in her dream.

———

Kelly had become too weak to lift his head or to verbalize his thoughts. Then the day before he died, his eyes shot open and he bolted forward in bed. Kelly's arms were outstretched with palms up to heaven.

That night his body became mottled, pulse disappeared and his watch stopped. Christy spent the night. At one point as she was leaning near, he forcefully grabbed her head, thrust it into his chest, and kissed her on the cheek. He waited to be alone with his wife before dying.

A few nights later, Kelly's mother Dee Dee Carman woke at 4:10 a.m. She saw Kelly's shadow. "Take care of Dad," was his admonition. Christy then "felt something tall behind me" as she was getting in bed. Dee Dee: "When someone dies, listen for the very soft fluttering of angel wings."

* * * * *

Katrina Pittman's mother was murdered. Even worse, Katrina secretly knew that her mother's boyfriend was the killer. But evidence was lacking. Katrina had strong Christian beliefs, but this was very unsettling.

Several days later Katrina heard it very audibly. It was her mother. She wanted Katrina to know she was OK. It was very reassuring.

‾‾‾‾‾‾

Katrina's Grandpa Mike had always loved horses. But Cupid was a horse dear to his heart.

Months after Gramps died, Katrina looked into Cupid's field longingly. She noticed Cupid was peaceful. Standing next to her was Gramps.

Her dead Gramps visits his horse

‾‾‾‾‾‾

Katrina sometimes sees those who have not transitioned. When walking through the hospital on her nurse's duties, she will glance in an empty room and see apparitions. In our office, often at the end of the day, she will look in the waiting room and see an older gentlemen sitting in a chair.

* * * * *

Leslie was heading home on a beautiful country road, bordered by horse farms. As she headed down a hill, she suddenly had a severe panic attack.

Never had Leslie panicked. She slowed the car to a crawl. Desperately, Leslie looked for a place to pull over to the side. Should she call her two sons? They would think she was crazy! How could she explain that she was suddenly too frozen to drive?

When starting up the next hill, Leslie was creeping at five mph. Suddenly a car crested the hill, passing on a double-yellow line in her lane. The panic attack averted a certain head-on collision and likely death. After Leslie's car topped the hill, her panic attack disappeared.

On arrival in Lexington, she called me. "Jim, you are the only one who would understand!"

* * * * *

In her adolescence, Tracy Harrod had an unfortunate experience. Her grandfather when drunk became inappropriate. Tracy's first marriage ended due to ongoing unfaithfulness, and the second when her child was mistreated. What was the use of trying? Tracy lost focus of what was most important in life. She turned to alcohol and cocaine.

One night Tracy had a vivid dream. Then suddenly she bolted up in her bed. Tracy felt a presence. It was her dead grandfather. She could feel his hand. Tracy even saw the indentation in the bed where he sat.

Her grandfather was not the silent type. "I'm going to kick your butt if you do not straighten out!" she audibly heard.

Her dead grandfather's visit

The language was unmistakable. She knew exactly what he meant. For her those words were full of love. She had heard them many times before. Her grandfather had come back to save her. Tracy has completely transformed her life. She has a strong knowing about God. Her daughter is contemplating a career as counselor or psychologist.

———

Tracy had known her best friend Peter since childhood. While in high school, Tracy dreamt Peter died in a car wreck. When she could not find him the next day, she fretted.

He had skipped school with his girlfriend Paula. That ended in a car accident. But he did not die.

Paula's father was furious. He told Peter he was sending his daughter away to a boarding school. "You will never see her again."

Peter was in shock. "Without her life is not worth living." He committed suicide.

This greatly upset Tracy. She has not dreamt since. In a school memoriam, they played an unforgettable Boyz II Men song.

Months later at a Western Hills High School beauty pageant she attended, they played that same song. Tracy suddenly felt cold. A hand brushed her forearm. Except no one was nearby. Then very distinctly she heard Peter's voice: "I'm OK. You can let go."

* * * * *

"I had been working the night shift at Kosair Children's hospital and only six months out of nursing school when one afternoon, I decided to take my eight-month-old Maltese puppy with me to pick up some lunch. She loved car rides.

It was a road I traveled often when suddenly approaching my vehicle, head on, was a beat up pickup truck coming straight towards my small Toyota. I turned to my right hoping I could pull off the road, but there was a large drop off. I surely would turn my car over if I chose that way.

In addition to feeling panicky, I realized I had my puppy on my lap. What would happen to her when the pickup hit us head on? All I could do was close my eyes and pray.

Immediately, I felt a huge presence envelop my puppy and I in place in the seat while the drunk driver plowed into my car head on. It was an overwhelming feeling of peace, calm and love like I've never felt before.

"I felt a huge presence envelope my puppy and I"

When the car came to a jolting stop, I opened my eyes to find the front end clear up to the windshield. Not a sliver of glass on me or my puppy. Ironically, the air bag never discharged which saved my puppy, still sitting on my lap, from being crushed.

The next scene in this chain of events was a furniture delivery truck driver tapping on my window to see if I was OK. The men were able to keep the drunk driver from fleeing the scene.

Fortunately, the furniture delivery truck had a cell phone, and this was a time when cell phones were not common (1993). The men called the EMS who arrived to help me out of the now tight enclosure of metal all around me. They lifted my dog through the side window, and she was perfectly fine. I was taken to the hospital to find only some bruises along my chest from the seat belt and a neck whiplash injury.

I survived what I feel was a near-death experience. Time stood still in that moment. Once the huge presence was all around and holding me, fear no longer existed. There was only complete love and acceptance. This event truly was the opening to my spiritual awakening and a complete knowing that we are not ever alone."

-Michelle Walden

Magical Midway

Angels, voices, visions and a friend sharing, "It is not your time." Yes, it is in your town, too! My small resort-like town of Midway, Kentucky is truly a very special place with "a church on every corner." I am blessed to be a part of a caring congregation with an outstanding, humble and loving minister.

Following her father's death, Beth Thompson was crushed. She became reckless. Beth drank alcohol every day of the following year "except for the days you can count on your hand."

At the start of the New Year, she began listening to the audio Bible. Soon she was praying. Her drinking ceased and life became focused. My fellow church member Beth then vividly dreamt of her father. He looked much younger and very healthy. Though Beth had questions as to whether she was following the right pathway, he smiled broadly. "Everything is alright."

* * * * *

She had always been taught to downplay pain. During childbirth, when asked how she was doing, Etta said fine. But she was not.

Staff suddenly took note. Things were not going well. They rushed into action. Meanwhile, Etta floated to the ceiling. Watching from above, she was in disbelief that the person below was truly her.

* * * * *

Marty was driving by a house when the house whispered to her. "Buy me, buy me." Later that day she again happened to pass the house. Once again it whispered, "Buy me." Marty fell in love with the house.

The house whispered, "Buy Me!"

When applying for a house loan, the preliminary loan officer told her she did not quite meet the criteria. Marty asked the loan officer to please pray for the loan to go through. It was days before Marty heard from the bank. She got the loan.

* * * * *

A terrible storm hit Jill's house in the country, shattering windows and ripping off a door. Years later when another frightening storm hit, Jill was in the laundry room panic-stricken. "God, give me courage!"

She reached into her dryer. Immediately landing in her hand was a piece of leather. It was inscribed with a single word: "Courage." Stashed in her purse, Jill never goes without it.

* * * * *

It was traumatic for Jack Morgan when he divorced his first wife. He dearly loved Charlotte, his new wife, who had become the salvation of his life.

Charlotte had a strong artistic gift. Their house was blessed with her colorful paintings hanging in every room. Charlotte too had generously painted wall hangings for her church. When her doctor disastrously painted a patient room a horrid green, she had a solution. She painted a magnificent mural that wrapped around the room, nicely depicting jungle animals and foliage.

The doctors were blunt. Charlotte had a life-threatening pancreatic cancer. Difficult surgery was performed, but it wasn't long before Jack began witnessing Charlotte's life slipping away. Then it did.

How he missed Charlotte! For Jack, life seemed no longer worth living. His very strong spiritual faith was fading. Where was God in his time of need? Why had God not saved Charlotte? Weeks passed.

Then months.

Jack awoke in the very early morning. Was it four a.m.? It was eerily quiet. In their neighborhood, normally dogs were barking, sirens blaring or at least the sound of cars could be heard passing. But not this night. It was dark and strangely serene.

Then Jack saw something at the foot of his bed. He squinted, but had difficulty making out details. It was a feminine figure.

He did not recognize her at first. She looked so healthy! A broad smile was on her face. Jack asked, "Are you an angel?" She responded in a way Jack immediately recognized. "No, but I'm working on it."

"Are you an angel?" "No, but I'm working on it."

It was his beloved. She reassured Jack that everything was fine. "God is love," she shared. Jack has basked in the sunshine she brought back into his life.

* * * * *

Catalina lost her first child at two years old. She and husband John were counseled that having a second was a big risk. They decided instead to adopt.

After connecting with a pregnant mother, they monitored her progress. But for Catalina something didn't feel right. They had nicknamed the baby Mick, for Michael. But Mick died at birth. Perhaps adoption was not best, Catalina thought.

One day when alone, she heard a distinct voice. "His name will be Luke." She rushed home to tell John.

GOD: "His name will be Luke"

Hours later the phone rang. Would it be too much trouble to come to North Carolina? They jumped at the opportunity, picking up their new adopted baby – Luke.

A year later, Catalina felt ill. She knew what the doctor would do. They would want a pregnancy test. Rummaging, she found an old kit. It tested positive. She was pregnant.

Emotions roiled. For the next five months, she and John worried. Would this child be sick? Would it die like their first?

Catalina birthed a strapping, boisterous baby boy, now a thriving toddler.

* * * * *

When giving birth, Libby Warfield declined drugs for pain. She wanted full awareness of her son's birth.

With her final push, she darted out of body. From her new perspective, she could watch her son emerging from her body. It was minutes after going back in body before Libby regained her breath.

———

Sitting on the porch of her sister's house, Libby was not sure. It seemed like a whisper, a faint voice from the upstairs window.

"Libby, Libby."

A faint voice whispered "Libby, Libby"

She thought her sister Peggy was playing a trick. When she looked through the window Peggy was lounging on the sofa with her dog.

Libby sat back on the porch. Again she heard, very clearly now, from the upper window. "Libby." Pause. "Libby."

She rushed to the door. Libby would intercept her sister before she got down the stairs. But there Peggy was, stretched out on the couch.

Three days later, her Aunt Grish tragically died. She had a stroke, fell against a furnace and died instantly. Libby knows the voice was a dead aunt warning her of the impending tragedy.

* * * * *

While in bed one night, Mike Perry had a heart attack. Everything went black.

On the other side, the smiling face of his dead 42-year-old cousin greeted him. "Boss" had previously died of a heart attack. Without speaking, Boss communicated, "You are not going to die." Others were behind Boss, but their backs were to Mike.

The smiling face of his dead cousin

It was a very peaceful experience. On awakening, Mike found himself on the floor. In the ambulance headed to the hospital, he felt remorse he had not died. It had been so wonderful.

* * * * *

When Anne Burford was a young girl, a small angel would visit. Periodically, she would see her resting on the doorknob.

One night after going to bed, her father stuck his head in to check on her. He was not expecting what he saw. Leaning over his daughter was an angel. Her wings were fully spread.

Her dad nearly tripped over himself as he rushed to grab his wife. The two then watched motionless, in awe. The angels never came back.

Her angel wings were fully spread

———

When a little older, Anne had a premonition about her brother Dennis. Brita told her parents that when the phone rings not to answer because something terrible had happened to Dennis.

The phone rang. Her dad answered. Dennis, he was informed, had been in a very bad car accident.

* * * * *

Missy every day checked in the barn on her llamas. What she found one day shocked her. "Carol Burnett" had U-shaped metal bars squeezing her neck. The bars were attached to a "muck" bucket. It was suffocating. Frantically, Carol Burnett tried to break free.

The llama was very tall. Melissa was short. She could not think. How could she help? She prayed. "God please help me. Help Carol Burnett!"

A calm, beautiful, succinct voice responded. "Get your elbow on top of Carol Burnett's head. Then push down."

Missy got on her tiptoes. She did not know how she could reach the top of the llama's head. Somehow she did. Quickly, Carol Burnett was freed.

Missy quoted Lily Tomlin: "Why is it that when we talk to God we're said to be praying, but when God talks to us we're schizophrenic?"

Lily Tomlin "Why is it that when we talk to God we're said to be praying, but when God talks to us we're schizophrenic?"

* * * * *

Though living in the country, Clarissa had stayed an intimate part of the small community where Eva Walters lived. Clarissa had been very excited about the birth of a baby, now six months old.

A violent summer storm hit on Clarissa's trip home from town. The road was thickly lined with trees that swayed powerfully with the wind. As lightning surrounded in all directions, a large limb snapped. It landed on Clarissa's car, killing her and the baby. Eva was anguished.

Months later, Eva celebrated her 16th birthday. Unexpectedly, she became ill. It was blood poisoning. The illness evolved rapidly. Soon Eva was in a coma.

Her parents became frightened and quickly summoned the town doctor. Somehow she heard her doctor share grim words with her family. Eva was going to die. Hovering above, Eva looked down at her parents and the doctor as the movie of her life unfolded.

Eva hovered above as the movie of her life unfolded

Suddenly, she was in a cave-like tunnel, very dark and long. In the far distance, she could see a tiny light. As it got closer, the light magnified. Its energy seemed very powerful.

In the distance, a woman became visible. Her shape was familiar. A broad smile crossed her face. It was Clarissa. "Eva, it is not your time to die." Quickly, Eva was back with her family.

My Incredible Mentors

Startling stories from my life's special guides from angels in many forms, a shocking surprise and admonition, and Jesus puts his hand into a chest to heal a heart.

The Angels Came For Him

My mentor, America's top botanical medicine expert, Donnie Yance: "I flew to Florida to see Shelley, my adopted father. Somehow felt I needed to go when I did. God had taught me to go with my intuition.

He had surgery, and they pumped him up on drugs, not herbs, and the food quality was lacking. He was in a rehab center. His body was shaking terribly and he was not eating much. They were medicating him, which did nothing to help with his anxiety and tremors. I tried to get some of my relaxing herbal formula into him, but was unable to.

I saw Shelley alive right after I got off the airplane and then he passed about six hours after that. At three a.m. my entire body broke into the most intense sweat I have ever had. Thirty minutes later, I got the call that Shelley had stopped breathing and was being rushed to the hospital. I believe this was the time he had begun to leave the world.

On my way to the hospital, they called to say he did not make it. I went to see him, be with him and pray over him. I was totally alone with him other than the angels that came and lifted his spirit from his body.

"Angels...came and lifted his spirit"

I prayed in my own words as well as recited all the appropriate

Christian prayers. I know he is not Christian, but I also know that it is what he would expect from me. He said thank you and looked so peaceful. I am happy for him because he never would have regained his physical or mental state to where he would want to be alive.

The next day while I was sitting outside Shelley's apartment, the most beautiful dragonfly landed on my arm and stayed there for a good two minutes. When a dragonfly lands on you, you will hear excellent news from someone far away from home. Represented in Japanese paintings, dragonflies are symbolic of new light and joy. To Native Americans, they represent a soul of someone who has passed.

Within my grieving and loss, I celebrate his life. I feel a sense of joy. Death is just a transition after all. He is resurrected and in his new body. We shall see him again. Cannot wait to hear his jokes again. I thank God for being able to be the last person with him and to help him transcend to the heavens."

* * * * *

A Shocking, Humorous Expression of God

One of Dwight McKee M.D.'s early clinical successes was with a lymphoma patient who was treated with radiation at Sloan-Kettering in the late 1970s, then told to "get her affairs in order" (chemotherapy for lymphoma had not yet been developed at that time). With intensive nutritional and mind-body therapies, she made a complete recovery and lived for 25 years after that. In the mid-1980s, her niece was presented with an even more aggressive (high grade) lymphoma than she had. Dwight worked with her as well, but she died from complications of chemotherapy in the hospital. Dwight was very upset and depressed by her death at 19 years of age.

Dwight's description of his mystical experience: "Several months after she had died, I got up from sleeping and went to the bathroom, then lay back down on my bed. Suddenly I heard a voice say, 'You must go back in the hospitals to teach compassion.' I looked around, and asked, 'For how long?'

A voice said "You must go back in the hospital to teach compassion"

The voice answered, 'Four years.' At this point, I said, 'Who is this?' As if to answer, I saw something come out of my ceiling that looked like a six foot long 'party favor' unrolling. Awesome energy seemed to be coming off the tip, and my body was vibrating on the bed. I said 'OK, OK.' It disappeared. I was definitely awake, eyes open, throughout the experience. Previously, I had toyed with the idea of going back into hospital training for oncology, but was not really serious about it. Subsequent to this experience, I made the decision to go back into hospital training: Three years of internal medicine residency, and three years of hematology/oncology fellowship. I hope I did some teaching of compassion along the way. It was the most dramatic mystical experience of my life, and definitely changed the course of it."

Dr. Dwight McKee is the number one integrative oncologist in America, who practiced holistic medicine and alternative cancer therapies for 12 years, and then trained in internal medicine, medical oncology and hematology, and practiced and taught integrative cancer medicine after training in hematology/oncology.

* * * * *

Jesus' Heart-Healing Hand

When Dean Ornish, M.D. wanted someone to direct his famous research on lifestyle and support in reversing heart disease, he called Lee Lipsenthal. Lee presented "The Science of Connection" at Bob's integrative holistic conference explaining how social connection is essential for health.

Lee also led an experiential group where I first glimpsed what heaven was like. With a strong musical beat playing in the background, one participant lies on the mat breathing deeply, another at their head to offers any needed support.

At one of these events, Lee witnessed an emergency. A man on a mat suddenly pressed his hands on his chest, gasping for air. Lee ran over to assist. It was quickly apparent that he was having a heart attack. He was dying.

Lee, feeling helpless, knew of only one thing to do. He prayed. Fervently.

Then it happened. Lee saw a hand on the man's chest. It penetrated through the chest. The hand appeared to grasp the man's heart.

A hand penetrated through his chest

Soon the man began to relax. His gasping subsided. Breathing returned to normal. Lee could hardly believe what he was seeing.

When trying to explain this later to his wife, she asked whose hand it was. Lee responded quickly. "It was the hand of Christ."

Lee's wife was hesitant to accept this explanation. Was he sure?

Lee, of Jewish heritage, said unequivocally, "Yes, it was Christ's hand. If you had seen it you would have known."

Lee died of esophageal cancer. This and other stories are included in his parting book, *Enjoy Every Sandwich*.

* * * * *

A Physician's Psychic Intuition

Bob Anderson, M.D., one of my mentors and founder of the American Board of Integrative Medicine, once mentored a student

Roscoe at his office before the major use of computers. Roscoe had typed out a term paper. He brought it strapped on the back of his motorcycle from home 60 miles away. On arrival Roscoe was panic-stricken that nearly all of the papers had flown away. He had no backup copy. For months he had worked on that paper.

Bob suggested they think on this calmly and meditate. As he did so, Bob visualized the papers along a steep slope of the interstate.

Bob visualized the papers

The two drove the 60 miles of interstate trying to identify the area. Fifty miles from the office, Bob spotted the steep slope. They stopped and searched. Quickly the papers appeared. Of the 73 pages, 69 were found.

* * * * *

A Luminous Ball from Heaven

Bob was sleeping soundly next to his wife one night in a nice Seattle suburb when a very bright glowing ball appeared outside their bedroom window that lit up the night. They were startled and confused by its appearance. What were their neighbors thinking?

They jumped out of bed. He went to check on the kids while his wife checked the house. Bob found the children sleeping soundly. When his wife got downstairs, she found that the iron had mistakenly been left on; the ironing board was smoldering and smoky. She rushed the ironing board out away from the house.

When they got back to their bedroom, the glowing ball had left. When they inquired with their neighbor who lived right next door and others across the street, they had not noticed anything. Bob shared this story with me personally and included it with other fascinating ones in his book, *Stories of Healing*.

* * * * *

The Mysterious Miracle Healer

Bob was so pleased when his son's wife gave birth to a fine baby boy.

He and his wife traveled to San Francisco to be with them.

The morning they arrived, the regular pediatrician was not in attendance. The doctor filling in gave a good report on the baby.

Quite unusually, the substitute pediatrician came back for a second visit midday. Concerns were raised, and a more extensive evaluation began. A spinal tap revealed life-threatening meningitis. Because of the quick diagnosis and aggressive management, the baby did well.

Mom and Dad followed up faithfully with the one-week visit at the office complex housing the pediatrician's office. The report was excellent. They were told to return again in a month.

When the two arrived for the second follow-up, they were surprised to find the office completely deserted. There was no sign of furnishings. When they asked at other offices in the complex, they were astounded to hear them claim no one had occupied that office for years.

The pediatrician and his office disappeared

How could their pediatrician have deserted them without a word? They had to know what happened! Checking with the hospital, there were no records by the doctor. In fact, no one with that name was on staff or registered by the state of California.

Bob's conclusion – it was an angel.

Mesmerizing Individuals

A Mother's Love from Beyond

AMY-This serious, intelligent, hard-working and generous woman comes from an outstanding family that is gifted in many ways.

"Easter has always been a special time for me. It's a time of deep reflection followed by renewed energy and vitality. The Easter of 2010, however, was particularly meaningful for me, and the experience would change my life forever.

The night before Easter I was preparing for bed. It was late and as I was trying to fall asleep I was overcome with a strange sensation. An unfamiliar feeling of urgency and anxiety swept over me. I then sensed an energetic presence in the room. It felt as if someone was standing at the end of my bed that I could not see, only sense. I felt the energy as loving and protective. As I was trying to make sense of things, a strong feeling came over me that there was something I needed to hear. There was a message that needed to be communicated.

Initially, I didn't know who was trying to contact me or even how or why this was happening. I just had the impression that I would not be able to rest until I figured out this message I was supposed to receive. I then heard a voice. Although I was startled, I listened. I was warned that my dad's health was in danger. Suddenly and without knowing how I knew, I had a strong feeling it was a blood clot. I then had a vision of my grandmother who had passed away when I was five. She was standing in her home and showed me a special memory I had as a child. My mind struggled for a moment to absorb what was happening. Then things started to make sense. My grandmother had come to send me a warning about my dad. As soon as I felt the message was heard, I relaxed and was able to sleep. As I was drifting off there was a strong feeling of peacefulness and a loving protective energy as if my grandmother was still with me.

"I then heard a voice"

Although my dad hadn't complained of feeling unwell, I called him first thing Easter morning. He is a serious man, reserved in expressing emotion. I was a little hesitant and unsure how he would respond. After telling my experience, there was a long pause. He finally stated, 'You described Grandma exactly as she was. I remember her working the late shift as a nurse. Even if I was already sleeping she would come in my room to check on me, give me a kiss, then would sit for awhile and watch over me.' He then choked up as he said, 'It is heartwarming to know my mother is still protecting and watching over me from the other side.'

"My grandmother had come to send me a warning about my dad"

The next day my dad scheduled a doctor appointment. His left leg had been a little sore lately, but he had presumed it was nothing serious. He was relieved when the doctor also felt it wasn't serious and advised him to put a heating pad on the area and no further testing was done.

Two days later, my dad came over for a short visit to play with the grandkids. Thirty minutes after he left, I was overcome with the feeling something wasn't right. It was almost like having a panic attack. I was pacing around and felt frantic, but had no idea why. Suddenly a stern voice commanded loudly, 'Call your dad.' Briefly I thought, 'I just saw Dad and he seemed fine.' I then saw a flash of light and the voice urgently repeated, 'Call your dad.' This time I didn't hesitate and I reached my dad as he was walking out the door to mow the lawn. Still feeling this sense of urgency I made him promise to rest tonight and see the doctor again tomorrow. I was insistent that he needed testing to rule out a blood clot. I was then able to relax and watch TV.

I started to smell perfume out of nowhere. I tried to figure out where the smell was coming from. It became so strong it was as if the bottle of perfume was right under my nose. Shortly after that I was putting my three-year-old son to bed. As he was brushing his teeth he said, 'Who keeps calling my name?'

A stern voice commanded, "Call your dad"

My husband and I looked around and said, 'We don't hear anything, let's get you to bed.' As we were tucking him in, he insisted someone called out his name, Christian, two times. The following morning Christian was busy playing with his trucks. He paused and called me over. 'Hey mom,' he said. 'Last night I met someone. She said her name is Grandma Marge. She's a nice lady.' I immediately called my dad to tell him what my son experienced. He was already back at the doctor's office. An ultrasound had revealed a large blood clot in his leg very close to the femoral artery. The doctor was now very concerned. The clot had the potential to break loose and could cause a life threatening condition. He was told to avoid strenuous activity and was started on two different medications to dissolve the clot. I was now relieved that my dad had a diagnosis. We were both under the impression that this was a close call that could have been deadly, but with treatment he would now be fine.

"Hey mom, last night I met…Grandma Marge"

The whole experience altered my life's direction. It peaked my interest in spirituality. Something prompted me to look into healing. Through a series of synchronistic events, I discovered an energy healing class that was offered that same week only five minutes away from my house. I took that as a sign and enrolled. I felt an immediate connection. Time seemed to fly by as I devoted myself to studying, taking more classes and practicing meditation.

One night as I was meditating, I felt the presence once again of my grandmother. I suddenly had a vision of my father. He was standing alone in the woods. Shortly after the vision, the now familiar energy and voice stated, 'Your dad is not out of the woods yet.' I fully trusted this time and called my dad right away. I again urged him to see the doctor and have another ultrasound. He also took this message quite seriously and scheduled the appointment. It was six months after starting the medication. The ultrasound showed the blood clot had not dissolved or diminished in size at all. I decided it was time to put my new healing skills to the test with my dad as my first client.

As I began our first session, I put my hands over the area of the clot. The entire area between his knee and hip felt energetically cold with no flow of energy to it. It felt like a large blockage. I heard a voice say, 'In four sessions, your dad will be healed.' We continued with weekly sessions, and each time I felt an improvement in the energy circulation to the area. On our fourth session, the area was pulsing with energy. For the first time I was able to see inside the body, almost like x-ray vision. Looking inside the vessel, I could see it was cleared of any blockage and had normal blood flow to the area. My dad decided to confirm my vision by ultrasound. It was another three months before he had one scheduled, but he insisted he have another right away. The ultrasound verified what I saw and felt. The clot was completely gone.

"...I was able to see inside the body almost like X-ray vision"

In the years since this experience, I have started a private practice and have helped many clients. However, I will always cherish my first energy healing and the loving encounter with my grandmother that led me to it."

-Amy Wadel

Angelic Dog "Tippy" and a UFO

MARILYN-A visit from a deceased dog, an angelic, prophetic warning and a UFO. If I were to go into the jungles of the Amazon, Marilyn would be on my team. Her "can-do" attitude, her forthrightness and powerful faith are beacons to all around her.

Marilyn Smedley was very close to her grandfather. At his graveside service, Marilyn saw his ghostly figure standing next to the minister. Hunched over before his death, her grandfather now looked younger and completely upright.

There was a second figure just behind him, who Marilyn thinks was her grandmother. She nudged her sister and asked, "Do you see that?" Her sister could only see a light next to the minister.

———

Marilyn's dog Tippy had many illnesses. He was at the vet frequently. Finally, Dr. Renneker said it was time for Marilyn to let go of Tippy. "We keep people from moving on. Dying people hang for a long time because their relatives are not ready to let them leave. They hold them back. We must let them go," Dr. Renneker shared. Marilyn strongly feels we can hold people and pets back, keeping them from dying.

Marilyn got another border collie, Christie, to replace her dear Tippy. Tippy had always been a close companion. The new dog, Christie, was wilder.

Once when cooking, Marilyn noticed Christie in the dog bed next to the stove. She was pleased. She felt it meant Christie would become a companion dog like Tippy.

Then she heard a scratching noise from the door. Christie was trying to get in the house.

She looked back. The dog on the bed had disappeared. She knows it was Tippy, who had come to let her know she approved of Christie.

Her beloved dead dog returns to visit

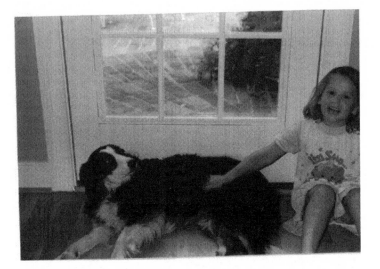

Marilyn was fascinated by mission trips to Colombia by her friend's sister Marty. "Marty, alert me of any opportunities to join you."

When Marilyn finished her nursing degree, the invitation was extended. They arrived at Bogota at night. When leaving the plane, armed guards surrounded them. It was clear they were not welcome. "I would have flown right back out if that was an option!"

No plans had been made for accommodations. Nothing was available. They had to settle for an area in the back of a bar. It was cramped, unsanitary with paper-thin walls.

When Marty unexpectedly announced she would be leaving for a few days, Marilyn felt vulnerable. A tall blonde American, she stood out.

She became extremely frightened. Finally, Marilyn realized the worst that could happen was rape, which she could survive, or death, leading to a positive spiritual afterlife. A strong sense of peace came over her.

She decided to leave immediately. She had to get to the U.S. Embassy across town.

Marilyn had to walk many risky streets to catch a bus. Walking with confidence, she succeeded.

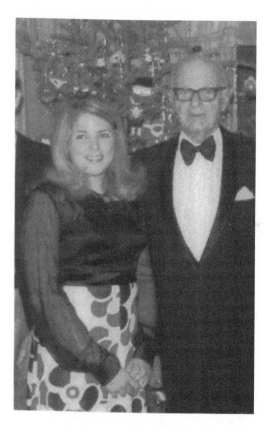

The bus dropped her at a sidewalk near the embassy. The street was open with no trees or other objects. No one was around. Yet after walking just a short way, she heard footsteps behind her.

Marilyn decided to immediately confront her stalker. Turning quickly, she shouted, "Why are you following me?"

It startled the short curly-haired, blue-eyed South American. Her first thought was, "He's not so big; I can take him!"

Nervously he said, "Don't go to the embassy today." Glancing and pointing at the embassy she said, "Well, it's just over there."

When she looked back, he had disappeared.

When she looked back, he had disappeared

Marilyn got the message. The bus had just turned around. She returned to the bus, certain the driver would think she was crazy.

On her way back into the city, she heard two explosions. It was the U.S. Embassy. She would have died.

Marilyn was driving I-75 in a rolling wooded area 30 miles south of Chattanooga heading north from Atlanta. Suddenly she noticed an expansive disc-shaped UFO hovering just above a forested area.

Her car mate was asleep. Marilyn tried to arouse her, but she was quite groggy.

When Marilyn looked back, the UFO was gone in a flash.

She knew many others on the interstate must have seen it. Marilyn stopped at the next gas station to hear the buzz about it. "What is being said about the UFO?" No one knew anything about it. When she checked the news, nothing was mentioned.

A Horse Ride to Heaven

MEGANN-Why our life matters! Are there horses in heaven? Can they help us transition? One story tears me up each time I read it. She is very special.

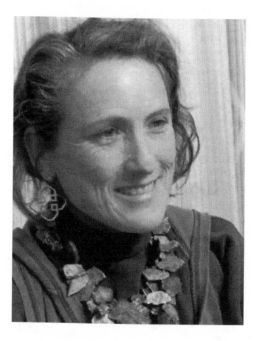

It begins at age eight on a family vacation in South Carolina. "I had lived six years with Type I Diabetes-insulin dependent. My control in those days was considered 'brittle' with many blood sugar highs and lows. It was still a time of ignorance by the medical establishment as how to manage this disease properly with food and injectable pig insulin. My mom helped me manage as best we could, never feeling confident about the next moment. Dad took all of my brothers on a day trip to see a military ship in the harbor, and Mom and I stayed at the condo. I had the flu and was put to bed for rest.

The next memory I have is of hovering above the room to watch a scene about to unfold. I see Mom check in on me when she noticed something was not right. Her action drew my attention to my own body across the room in bed, but I was not in it. My body had gone into an extremely low blood sugar reaction and I was convulsing.

Mom had educated herself on every aspect of my care and knew what to do. This was a fairly common occurrence. I watched from the opposite corner of the ceiling as Mom rushed to feed orange juice and liquid glucose to my shaking body.

Floating, I felt no emotion; there was just awareness of what was happening. There was no judgment or even fear. I reached out for Mom and she was next to me on the bed, but I could not seem to reach her. She was next to me, but at the same time seemed 50 feet away.

Suddenly, I felt juice flow into my mouth as Mom coaxed me to swallow. 'You can do it Megann, just swallow, my love,' she said firmly as I could now see the concern on her face. I was back. I could feel Mom's touch and the weight of my physical body.

Bewilderment seized me. I knew this experience was special, but not wanting more concern or attention focused in my direction, I pretended to be as normal as possible. After that experience as a child about which I never spoke, I felt myself turning inward. The world did not seem to make sense to me. Television shows made me cry, as they always seemed to exploit the weak and encourage the violent. I struggled to feel joy and love in my life. I felt burdened and heavy like the weight of the world was on my shoulders. I was insecure and self-conscious because people around me did not seem to see the sadness I experienced in the world.

As I grew into my teens and then young adulthood, the feelings intensified into a deep depression. I looked to artificial means to lift my spirit with no results. In fact, my life took a nose dive resulting in diabetic complications including blindness, heart disease, lethargy, neuropathy, digestive issues, kidney disease and weight gain.

Eventually in my 30s, I had a heart attack. My heart had been slowly breaking my whole life and finally it gave way. This single event was to change my life forever. After a month of cardiac rehab, I returned home overwhelmed by thoughts of dying. I sat on my porch looking out at the farmland around me wondering what my purpose was.

As I began to sob, I consciously realized there was no sound. Looking at the wind in the trees and the birds singing in the branches, I was completely deaf. A voice spoke as if in my head, but clearly out loud and said, 'You must do the best you can with what you have.' As soon as my hearing left, it was back. The wind in the trees rustling the leaves was like an orchestra with the bird's song the choir. My senses had returned, but the experience left me wondering whether I might not have only had a heart attack, but now I was going insane.

GOD: "You must do the best you can with what you have."

In the following months, I had many more intuitive and spiritual experiences which included 'seeing' the newly departed. As people I had known growing up died, they visited me while I showered. I had four waking visions that included important messages.

For privacy I will not use names, but the first individual showed me a picture of the voyage for one that is not spiritually connected. She appeared with a grey face looking long and drawn. Like a dramatic scene from the movies, she pointed to a winding road behind her on which many souls traveled. Each with a similar expression, much like the famous Edvard Munch painting, *The Scream*. The road wandered off into the distance toward the horizon with seemingly no destination. Each soul looked to be in deep concentration reliving the decisions of their life. My friend turned and joined the travelers on the road with shoulders rolled forward as if carrying a great burden. As I watched I noticed an energy, like a hand, would appear in the sky carefully and gently scooping individuals up off the path then together vanishing from sight.

A grey face, long and drawn. Souls with an expression like "The Scream"

The second individual who visited was not yet departed. It was Easter morning. Her body looked divided down the middle. One side old and sick, while the other young and well. Her message, 'I am half in this world and half in the next,' was meant for her family who was leaving on vacation. She had been sick for many years battling cancer, and I do not believe her loved ones knew the extent of her illness. She wanted me to tell them this message, but I was afraid of reaching out and their reaction. I refrained. She died two days later, during the family's vacation. I vowed at that moment never to be afraid of sharing such information even at the risk of others misunderstanding.

The third individual who visited in less than six months was a woman I had known and loved since I was a child. She was diagnosed with aggressive cancer and given a poor prognosis with only several months to live. When she passed, she also visited a day later after her death. She showed up not in the shower, but sitting in a chair at my kitchen table. Her youthful, vibrant face was full of joy and life. She asked me to give her sister a message: 'Tell her that I am well, out of pain and full of love.' I turned my gaze to a distraction in the room and when it returned she was gone.

In her seat was another familiar soul. A woman from the 1800s I had only known through pictures. She had been raised in the house in which I resided. She said nothing, but smiled as if to reassure me in her graceful mothering manner. What struck me most as I reflected was the strength and constitution of the two women. Love surrounded them and their hearts felt pure. I had the feeling they were gifting me with a part of their strength and vitality.

With the promise I had made to deliver messages to whom they were intended, I set off to find my friend's sister. I never even knew she had a sister so I went to visit her best friend. As you can imagine, words eluded me, but her friend listened patiently to my story without judgment. When I finished my story, big tears welled up in her eyes and she said, 'Well....I am her sister. Even though she has a real sister, she always told me I was her sister. The message was meant for me.'

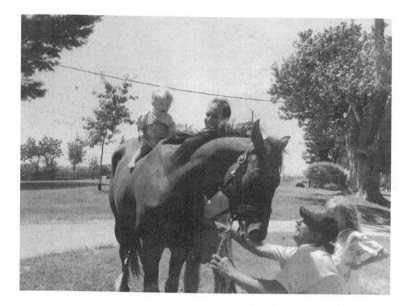

The last in this series of visits came from a very unexpected place and involved two souls. A young woman I knew who grew up near my farm took her life. I had seen her just weeks before and showed her my newly born baby goats. I let her hold one in her arms, and she had smiled as she cuddled it like a baby. She often walked down to visit my horses and feed them treats. Her favorite was my retired thoroughbred Tumble who with anticipation watched over the fence for her visits.

I did not know she had taken her life for half a day as I was dealing with my own animal family tragedy. I was dealing with my own grief. While attempting to load Tumble on a trailer, he reared up and back hitting his head on the metal support frame of the door. In his distress, he reared again and fell backwards landing on his spine, breaking his neck. He was paralyzed from the neck down and had to immediately be put to sleep. When I learned about the suicide I was shocked and heartbroken…but God is so good because there was a connection between the two horrific events I would soon realize.

Preparing for the visitation of the young woman, I stepped into the shower. The vision came in bold and clear. My dear horse was there in his full glory prancing with joy and vigor. He had come to escort the young woman on her journey to the other side. She appeared as a little girl not more than seven with long flowing hair and a beautiful yellow dress. She was thrilled to see him and climbed on his back, which was adorned with white flowers. Together they rode into the sunset as if they were one.

"My dear horse escorted the young woman to the other side"

In light of these almost unbelievable experiences, I have devoted myself to understanding psychic phenomena and their spiritual connection. In western culture, much has been lost of our spiritual nature, but in the indigenous cultures of the world such visions are viewed as precious gifts filled with important information. Spiritual awakenings are both healing our bodies and reconnecting us to our purpose in this life. Each of us has an important purpose, which many never find. It seems our purpose or our passion becomes obscured by a society based in artificial ideas of perfection and ruthless commercialism. Our spiritual nature, our Soul, is profound and abundant. It is the place from which all true healing emerges.

Over the last several years I realized I was neither insane nor broken. The understanding and support 'tools' I had searched for my whole life have been found by studying Energy Medicine and Energy Psychology. The health of our spiritual body, our energy body, our spiritual nature, our soul or whatever you want to call it, is as important to our physical bodies as the precious nutrients we eat, the air we breathe or the water we drink."

-Megann Thomas

Dead Visitors

The lively PIKEVILLE DUO are connected to the Beyond. These spiritual women would be among the first to stand up for their friends. Their deep roots in faith and understanding of our connection to "the other side" magnify their magnetic personalities.

God appears to Rita in her dreams as four to six beams of light. Then she hears a spiritual, echoing voice. She knows what is ahead. A family member will die. Rita awakens with a heavy feeling on her chest. That "weight" remains until the death of the family member.

———

Rita, a stage performer, had a family that kept news of illness secret. A voice in her dreams would tell Rita to call home. Nine out of 10 times, a family member had a serious illness.

In a dream on Christmas Eve, Rita was told her mother would die. In the dream, her mother's casket was white with beautiful flowers. After that dream, Rita hummed a sad religious song. Surprisingly though, she was upbeat. Per family tradition, she told no one. Two months later, Rita's mother died. On his own, her brother picked a white casket. With flowers, the sight was identical to her dream.

———

Rita and her husband grieved when her only pregnancy ended in miscarriage.

Many years later, her husband Jake developed cancer involving the brain. As death neared, he was delirious for four days. The night before he died, Jake awoke at 2:10 a.m. He was glowing.

"Honey, guess where I'm going. I'm going to see our baby!"

———

Grandfather Ben knew literally every word of the Bible. He had read it 21 times. "When Dad replaced our floor, he found on the floor joist an old maroon Bible dated 1889." It was accidentally left there during construction. The family Bible was inscribed by her great grandfather.

Shortly after Rita's Grandfather Ben died, her grandmother said one morning, "I saw Pappy last night!" She had a glow. There was a tall shadow next to her. Her grandmother said, "Shhh. God's here."

———

"God told me to get a one-year-old female teacup poodle," Rita shared. Her husband Jake was exasperated. "I'll give you a $1000 if you don't get one!"

Rita called her sister who had an animal kennel. She had a teacup poodle, but it was not female or a year old. But her sister did finally locate the exact teacup poodle.

It has brought her so much joy. Jake even fell in love with it. They ended up getting two more!

Jake died on Oct. 29th. The next day the dog went down the hall to her husband's picture. She would not take her eyes off of the picture until she fell asleep that night. Rita knows the dog detected her husband's presence with the picture. The next day, the dog returned to normal.

Rita's dog detects her dead husband

* * * * *

Once Bobbi saw an angel, appearing as a Spanish woman in plain clothes. Bobbi felt her positive energy. The angel was looking at the bar. A book appeared on the bar. It was the book Bobbi was writing, but had not finished. The book had the exact title she was planning to use. The cover was exactly the one she had envisioned. When she looked back, the angel had disappeared. When she returned her gaze to the bar, the book had disappeared.

The book is titled *Karma*. It reveals the rewards of good karma, but is frank about the costs of negative karma.

Angel to Bobbi: Finish your book!

Years after her father died, her mother remarried. Her mother had spent time at Bobbi's house while her stepfather was still alive. Months after his death, Bobbi saw a shadow walk from the bedroom to a closet, most likely her stepfather. "She doesn't live here anymore," Bobbi informed him. That was the last she saw of the shadow.

Bobbi knows she has visiting "ghosts." From time to time, her keys or jewelry will be found misplaced. She tells the ghosts, "Stop fooling around!" Usually within 15-20 minutes she locates her lost items.

They will make distracting noises. "You are making too much noise, you need to leave!" she would reprimand and it would quiet down. Dead pets are also frequent visitors.

When Uncle Cliff came to visit, he sat down in a favorite chair and turned on a halogen lamp. Bobbi never liked that light, as it got too hot. After he died, she came home one evening to find the halogen light on. She knew her Uncle Cliff had been to visit.

Spirituality Teaches Fearlessness

NESS has no fear. Unpretentious, extremely considerate and uplifting, he emphasizes the positive. He trusts in God and loves humanity. He has a level of kindness rarely found in a man.

When he was seven years old, Ness (Naser Alamdari) liked to tease his older cousin Mina. One morning when she was in a deep sleep, Ness poked her side. Furious, she chased him all over the yard. When Mina finally caught him in her rage, she choked him and then threw him to the ground lifeless.

Ness was floating above looking down. He felt the best he has EVER felt. Ness saw his spirit as a faint, white, transparent color. He could see in any direction with just a slight turn of his head.

Ness's spirit was a faint, translucent color

His older sister yelled. Ness could see Cousin Mina sobbing. His Aunt Lena in the kitchen ran out alarmed. Ness felt sorry for all three. Aunt Lena pinched his rectum. Ness felt his spirit being sucked back into his body. "No, no, no!" he exclaimed.

———

Ness's father died of lung cancer. Less than 48 hours later, 6000 miles away, Ness was awakened by his dad's energy. Near the door he could see the upper half of his dad. He was wrapped in a white robe. "Papa, papa!" His dad smiled. He had no teeth. His face was white as a ghost. Then he vanished.

On the fourth year after the death of a loved one, it is tradition to visit their grave. Ness flew to Turkey for the occasion. Afterwards, when everyone had left except his mother, Ness sat down with her. He learned that in the final weeks of his father's life he was not able to use or feel his legs. Ness asked about his teeth; his father wore dentures, his mom said. It is Islamic tradition before burial to remove everything from the body – all jewelry and dentures. Before burial, you are wrapped in a white cloth. Ness had asked about his father's paleness. "Yes, he was very pale at the end of his life."

———

His niece's fiancé committed suicide. Three years later, the fiancé appeared in Ness' dream. In the dream, he took Ness to an area of the Red River Gorge with a cave and other distinct features.

Ness told his niece Ann who was disbelieving. The two followed the way he had been shown in his dream to the exact spot of the cave. "It was his private cave where he liked to retreat," she shared.

Ness' dream told him of a fiancé's cave at the Red River Gorge

Ann is dependent on serious prescription drugs. The dead fiancé is not ready to leave until "she is situated."

———

Ness senses the impending death of relatives. "It comes to my soul." When alerted, he will call his family home in Turkey. Twice he learned close relatives had died in the previous few days.

———

Since his near-death experience in childhood, Ness is fearless. There is no concern of death. He doesn't mind working high on scaffolding. He walks along the edges of cliffs.

Recently, there was a terrible wreck on the interstate. Many stood around watching as a car burned with a woman inside. Ness broke through the glass and pulled her to safety.

Ness pulled a woman from a burning car

Ness assumes God will not take him until it is his time. His intuitive gifts all began after his near-death experience.

Miraculous Healing Through Prayer

LYNN is a very kind, educated woman who is the essence of spirituality in her demeanor and interactions. Lynn exemplifies miraculous healing through prayer. She is someone you could always count on in time of need. Conquering a fatal disease in her humble manner has inspired physicians and others. Her bond with spiritual healer Rosemary has produced many positive outcomes.

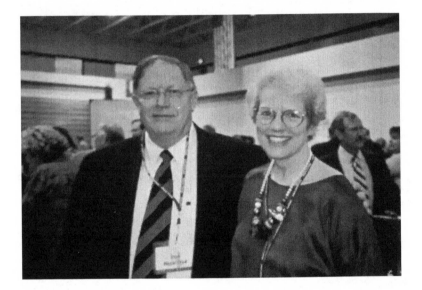

An educator and well spoken, Lynn Beck upheld exemplary standards. But something was happening to her health, which was worsening. From what began as a thin frame, she had lost 70 lbs. and was often losing consciousness. Doctors couldn't explain this until she saw an infectious disease specialist who discovered she had end-stage AIDS. Unknowingly, she had contracted HIV from an improperly sterilized needle in a physician's office.

With that diagnosis came the report that she had Cryptococcal meningitis, a disease with only a two percent survival rate. Her doctor explained that, with these issues and a destroyed immune system, there was no hope.

Lynn's husband, Stan, then sent many requests for prayer. At a church service in the next county, 80-year-old Margaret, a known prayer warrior heard that request. She said that God told her to pray for Lynn's complete healing. Although she didn't know Lynn, she found her address and began sending encouraging messages, complete with scriptures from the Bible.

Several years later, Lynn was invited to speak to a prayer group at Margaret's church and thankfully met Margaret for the first time. After that meeting, Margaret held a healing prayer session for those in need. Lynn then heard others tell their healing stories as a result of Margaret's prayers. For example, a young man with a brain tumor reported healing, after the doctors said it was untreatable.

Years later, Lynn's doctor said her recovery was remarkable and that he thought it was God. When Lynn said thanks to you and God, her doctor replied, "No, it was only God."

Her doctor: "No, it was only GOD"

Rosemary, a neighbor, who has a ministry of healing, came to see Lynn and offer prayer for God's healing energy. She explained to Lynn that she didn't accept money for her work since it was a gift from God. But she always suggests paying it forward by helping someone.

Once when visiting Rosemary, she surprised Lynn when she said, "You can't raise your right arm." When Lynn asked how she knew this, Rosemary replied, "I can feel your pain. It is because of unforgiveness. When you can forgive, your arm will heal." And that's exactly what happened.

Rosemary believes strongly in prayer as a supplement to her treatments. Occasionally when Lynn is not busy, Rosemary asks her to set aside a specific time to pray.

Rosemary was treating Janice, whose husband James was not a believer. He stayed in the next room while Rosemary treated his wife. When James came in after the treatment, Rosemary thanked him for praying for Janice. Startled, James asked how Rosemary knew that. "I just know." She always senses when others are praying for clients during treatment.

Rosemary senses others prayer

－－－－－

When a Qigong master used by Mayo Clinic came to town, Lynn went to listen. It was so intriguing she asked for a private session.

Her daughter, who was pregnant, called in tears; she had incapacitating hives. Lynn asked the Qigong master for solutions. He said the problem is in her liver.

Lynn asked, "Doesn't liver represent anger?" He said, "No, it's fear." When she went to the doctor, blood tests confirmed a liver issue.

－－－－－

Lynn's son had a severe 60-degree curvature of the spine. Surgery was necessary. The most his doctor hoped for was a 30-degree improvement.

As Lynn prayed, she saw a vision of her son walking toward her with his back straight and surrounded with blue light. Blue light, she later learned, is a color of healing.

During the twelve-hour surgery, she waited confidently. When completed, the surgeon was surprised. He had corrected the spine dramatically, leaving only an 18-degree curvature.

－－－－－

When Lynn was ill with AIDS, she encountered Bill, who had very advanced cancer. Bill's close and extended family had prayed dutifully up to that point. But the cancer had reached such a hopeless state that he knew they had given up. Bill shared this with Lynn, who said she would pray for him, and this she did fervently.

Weeks later in the middle of the night while Lynn prayed for Bill, a golden light appeared in each of her hands. What did this mean?

A golden light appeared in each hand

The special lights stayed on her hands for a long time. Then suddenly, they disappeared. She noted the time on her clock. Minutes later, Lynn received a phone call. Bill had died. She wanted to know when he had died. The time of his death was precisely when her hands had stopped glowing.

———

Lynn's gift and purpose was to encourage, she had always felt. But once when meditating Lynn heard a voice say, "You will appreciate."

When reflecting on this, her son had an explanation. Encouragement is speaking to others. Appreciating is listening to others.

———

Lynn's neighbor had a baby girl, but before a year old, it was diagnosed as blind. As they returned from St. Louis, with her husband driving, Lynn stretched out in the back seat. She prayed continuously that the baby regain sight.

Driving through downtown Louisville, Lynn saw something outside the car window. It looked like a white dove flying alongside the car. She could not believe her eyes. She asked her husband if he saw anything.

A white dove flew alongside the car

"Yes, a white bird. I think it is a dove."

Lynn was overcome with a strong sense of peace. She intuited it as an affirmation of her prayers.

When told about the experience, the baby's mother was puzzled. Repeatedly she asked, "What does it mean?"

Soon, the baby was retested. Her eyesight was restored.

A Unique, Harrowing "Kundalini"

MARLA excitedly and humbly shared an awe-inspiring, dangerous transformation that she learned is a "Kundalini" experience. Energy rises from the root chakra to the top of the head resulting in mystical awakening. The Higgs-Boson "God" particle field gives mass to any energy traveling through it. Is what Marla visualizes a "raw" picture of God?

Marla attended a Catholic school until entering a public arts program, followed by a conservatory, so she had a strong arts background. As she was more open-minded, "I was shown things." She recalls learning, "Before enlightenment, chop wood, churn water."

In researching her experience, she "found things I had seen in the multiverse (multiple universes)." During the experience, "I found things I KNEW I had not known before. It was a psychedelic experience, but I had not taken psychedelics. It was so intense. At the time I was in a dark period, having left everything - my community and network of friends. My work environment had been toxic. I moved seeking healing and peace. There were no buffers to the world. I was in a raw place. Post-traumatic stress syndrome was diagnosed.

I started meditating a lot, initially at the end of yoga. Mathematical binaural beats were used to induce brain waves. I ate a raw organic diet, drank macha and took ashwagandha, shatavari and tulsi tea.

Eastern people work with a master who guides them through kundalini experiences, but when you do it your own way it is very scary. You should not mess with the spiritual world. You can awaken yourself prematurely. It is very violent and scary. I was stunned. I was stripped of all padding that had separated me from spirituality.

"You should not mess with the spiritual world…it is very violent and scary"

Afterwards, I had a very intense feeling of creating reality all of the time. People can have too much electricity from the universe and completely lose it. It is important to ground yourself. You feel like a floating head. It is intense."

Marla's description: "In November of 2013, I had an uncontrollable out-of-body experience, whereupon right before sleep I shot straight out of my body and into the spiritual realm, for lack of a better explanation. Truly, I was ejected from my body. It was very intense. It began with a low vibration that increased in frequency and intensity, and resulted in a powerful ejection from this physical plane, in which I seemed to be electrically launched into another dimension or dimensions.

During my flight through the cosmos, but not the cosmos as we know it - rather, the cosmos in all of its multiversal bounty - I encountered 'the grid,' envisioned myself as living many different lives simultaneously and saw all of existence as projections of light. It was a beautiful, profound experience.

"I envisioned myself living many different lives simultaneously"

Up to that point, I had been an atheist. The experience culminated in mounting fear and anxiety at the intensity of my journey, and so I chose to 'find God' (literally) for protection. And 'find God' I did.

I ended up simply being in a non-space where a huge electrical generator was streaming forth thoughts (ephemeral pre-existent non-objects, they seemed like). I spent a long time in this 'space,' which at the same time seemed like a void, not a space at all. Perhaps I spent a very short time there, maybe 15 minutes or less. Regardless, it felt like eons had passed, and also only like I'd just blinked my eyes. I felt comforted, warm, safe and exalted. It was the singularly most profound experience of my life to date, bar none.

I almost chose not to return. However, a loud, insistent knocking brought me to a place of fear, and the fear brought me shooting back into my body. I do not know who was knocking or why. To this day, I do not know.

When I awoke, I realized my little black cat was sitting right next to my head, protectively guarding my physical body. After that experience, my relationship with my cat has transcended quite a bit, but that is another story altogether.

"My little black cat was sitting right next to my head protectively"

For many nights following what I believe was a traditional Kundalini Awakening, I had to practice the 'grounding technique' of gripping a coin that my mother gave me depicting a guardian angel. This 'grounding' kept me from subsequent ejections from my body. For several weeks following the initial astral projection of the awakening of Kundalini energy, the low vibration would begin as I started to fall asleep each night, increasing in intensity, until, by gripping the coin and feeling its physicality, I was able to bring the 'astral engine' to a slow stutter, and stop it altogether.

After some research, I discovered the Higgs-Boson. I saw that it was sensationalized as the 'God Particle,' although many scientists do not agree with that term, and it does not accurately describe the particle in real terms. Regardless, I was shocked by the photos of the Higgs-Boson, as they were exactly what I had seen when I 'went to God.' The two circles, with the vast electrical light projections streaming forth, were the exact depiction of what I had seen during my out-of-body experience.

Today, I believe I had been in a 'space' (even though this does not accurately describe where I was) with Brahma, or the Creator God. I now believe in the Christian Trinity, and the Hindu Trinity of the Godhead.

"The Higgs-Boson was exactly what I saw when I went to GOD"

I am currently a very religiously spiritual person who practices daily meditation, prayer, yoga and an Ayurvedic lifestyle, and consider myself a progressive, New Age Christian. I attend Unity Church and am grateful to be in the company of like-minded individuals."

A Vivid Second Near-Death Encounter

NASHID (KOLEOSO)-Two near-death experiences and a worldwide search for answers. Nashid – whose spiritual name is Koleoso - is one of the most incredible individuals of many I have met on this journey and a close friend. His death experiences and worldwide spiritual exploration transformed this rebellious young man into a sage. He speaks more eloquently about spirituality than anyone I have ever heard. His spirit and truth powerfully radiate from his soul.

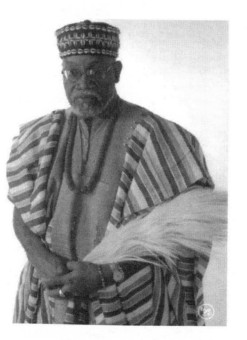

African tradition holds that major life developments occur every seven years. At age 21, the spiritual eyes flicker. Koleoso when 21 went to Okinawa in 1968, serving as a medic in the Armed Forces. It was a restless time and he was rebellious.

One day he had to deliver supplies. He whipped around a dirt road and lost control. Koleoso plowed into a building, which if he had missed, would have led to an 80-foot plunge into the ocean.

Koleoso traveled through a tunnel into the white light. The experience there was indescribable, unconditional love. He was told, "It's not your time yet."

Koleoso was completely transformed. He was hungry to learn more. He studied every religion. He settled on the Imam community in Michigan, yet while they said many of the right things, he did not feel the spirit behind it.

In 1978, Koleoso was very conflicted. He met a yogi in India who took up a special interest in him. When they ran into each other, the yogi always asked him to come over. Koleoso did not understand why he would be interested in an arrogant African-American.

He would just sit with the Yogi. The Yogi without conversation could read his past lives. He was able to communicate telepathically. The Yogi told Koleoso the problem was not the religion, but him. Koleoso was introduced to Sufism, which was more aligned with his beliefs.

The yogi without conversation could read his past lives and communicate

His faith wavering, Koleoso wanted a more concrete connection with God. He then asked God for "the reality of him." This he received.

Days later a car crossed four lanes of traffic and hit him head on. His nose was nearly severed off. He had broken so many bones in his face that his X-ray report was two and a half pages long.

During the accident, Koleoso was immediately thrown into a near-death state. He felt like he was in a void and incredibly vulnerable. It was as if he was bound to a chair naked in the middle of New York City. He could not get under it, could not get around it. Koleoso sensed he was being asked how he could ever doubt God. He knew he was being told that this could never happen again.

He felt like he was bound to a chair naked in the middle of New York City

He saw a gray cloud with faces representing all of the good and bad he had done in his life. Then he felt as if he was traveling down a river. On the right, a group of individuals approached up to the edge that he intuited were his ancestors. They observed him and then left.

There was much scurrying about. He felt the presence of an entity. Koleoso knew he was in the presence of "the power of powers." "Christ was with me."

In the presence of the power of powers

He had the sense of all knowing. Every question was immediately answered. Koleoso recognized we are all one with the universe. Like a drop in the ocean, we are all one and all powerful. It had been dark, but then a light arose on the horizon. It got warm. He felt an immense sense of pure, unconditional love.

Ever since, Koleoso has spent his life searching for the meaning of this. He communicates with entities that guide him.

He had gone to law school. But Koleoso has come to realize that he is to promote the law of God. Today, people are mainly feeding their sensibilities, which is OK. But it is the little things that are important, the small acts of kindness. We must initiate the young; if we do not initiate them, as African saying goes, they will burn down the village just to feel the heat.

Shamans read signs. When the wind shifts, it means the wind is with you. One hawk has positive implications. When you see two hawks though, there will be a challenge in three days. Kidney disorders mean you are too serious. Heart problems signal a lack of love.

In his studies, Koleoso has discovered the strong similarities between near-death experiences and what transpires in the initiation ceremony for shamans.

Shaman initiation mirrors near-death experience

Both in current indigenous tribes, and back in our history when tribal cultures were predominant, shamans served as the liaison between God and the tribe. They were usually individuals that we would consider misfits in today's society. Some had seizure disorders, or might today be considered schizophrenic, but were highly regarded in those tribes and served a true healing purpose.

This principle is consistent with what I have discovered clinically, that those who have had special challenges in their life, especially during childhood, are given a compensatory spiritual gift.

Koleoso wrote a book *The Near Death Experience: A Vehicle of Shamanic Initiation*, focusing on the similarity between spirituality gained from the near-death experience and becoming a shaman.

———

I asked Koleoso if he would pray for a trip I was making to New York City to meet with the media.

He pulled out some aged felt cloth in which cards were wrapped. Koleoso spread the cards out evenly, overlapping, facedown and proceeded to tap over them four times with his knuckles. He would then pull out a card, then repeat the process a total of four times.

He then looked at each card individually and said that all four said that my trip to New York would go very well and that I would be well-received. I thanked him. My trip indeed went very well and has had a strong influence on my life journey. I find that there are an infinite variety of ways that truly spiritual people can tap into the spiritual realm. It does not mean that everyone using these techniques is a spiritual person.

———

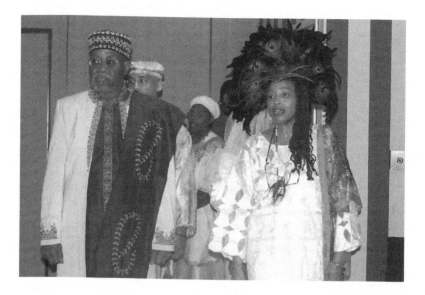

Osunnike had been living in Boston practicing her intuitive and alternative healing work, and then moved to Jamaica to continue that work. While there, she developed a severe fibroid tumor condition and felt compelled to come back to Boston for treatment.

While back in Boston, Osunnike connected in with a group of other alternative healing practitioners that set up a website chat line. Koleoso, who she did not know, had joined the website, and one day posed a question about healing work. She was the only one that answered. Subsequently, they e-mailed back and forth.

She felt an old and familiar attraction to Koleoso. He asked her to come to Kentucky to heal his wife who had been ill for many years. Osunnike was torn over whether to go, as she knew his wife and children's mother's health was declining and she required his constant attention.

She then had a premonition that told her not only to go, but also to refuse payment. There was something else about this journey that was compelling her to go. Yet, she could not understand this as she hardly had any money of her own at this time. But she obeyed and went.

After arriving she felt very strongly drawn to Koleoso, but knew he was fully devoted to his wife's care. It would be very important to honor the integrity of their marriage and not interfere or be a burden. But she could not shake these familiar feelings and closeness.

Finally, after a very intense and powerful healing week with Koleoso's wife, Osunnike decided it would be best to go back to Boston and not look back. However, to her absolute amazement, his wife asked her to stay and become a part of their family.

This was amazing and because Osunnike had become so close to Koleoso during her stay there, she decided to share with him one of her most powerful past life regressions of an extremely important lifetime she had in Egypt. As she was telling him the story, to her amazement, he finished it for her. She had been a high priestess whose spiritual calling was to oversee the King and his harem. And yes, Koleoso knew from his own past life remembrances that he had been that King.

As she was telling her Egyptian past life experience, he finished it for her

Miraculous Healings, Ghosts and Mystery

BRUCE-A gentle, passionate Christian with remarkably diverse and unique experience, when he presented at our Sunday School class, we were captivated. Bruce has an impressively strong faith and speaks from his heart.

Bruce's mother was sick with metastatic colon cancer. He was in Georgia when he felt the urge to return to Kentucky to be with her. Bruce sped in his car, passing three state troopers in Georgia, three more in Tennessee and finally three in Kentucky. He was clearly speeding, but they paid no attention to him.

"When I said to my mother, 'It's Bruce, I'm home from Georgia,' she opened her eyes, placed hers upon mine with those beautiful piercing eyes. I said to her, 'I know and I love you too. You've been such a precious loving mother and I love you so much. You have been living your whole life to one day be with Jesus. Now you go on and I'll see you later.' I moved her eyes and she let out her last breath."

After her death, she came back to him one night while he was in bed to let him know that she was OK. Bruce hugged her and then she vaporized.

His mother came back a second time when he was in a very negative relationship that had brought him way down. When she appeared, he knew why she was there. Bruce immediately broke off the relationship.

Before Bruce's mother had died, she had been in a Lexington hospital with her cancer. While at her bedside, he saw her leave her body accompanied by a bright light that he recognized as angels. It was a good while, likely many hours, before she returned.

He saw her leave her body, accompanied by a white light

Later Bruce asked her about what she experienced while she was out of her body. She looked at him with very piercing eyes that said, "I know I left my body, but how did you know?" She finally said it was her experience, and it was not appropriate for her to share it with him.

———

One day, Bruce and his wife were driving through Versailles. He had a major knee problem. Walking was difficult. He was turning left off of Main Street to head toward the bank branch. Instead, his car wheel pulled strongly to the right. It turned Bruce and his wife down a side street. They were headed to Big Spring Park.

When they arrived, his sister Priscilla was there, who Bruce calls a "prayer warrior." She had been praying for his arrival. She performed a "laying on of the hands" as she prayed fervently for him.

Afterward, Bruce and his wife drove home. He got out of the car and was walking toward the house when his wife yelled, "Honey! Do you see what you are doing? You are walking normally!" To this day, his knee is completely healed.

———

The next youngest son, "Cheeseburger," dropped an iron on his right eye, severely burning it. They rushed to the Emergency Department to get help.

Bruce's mother asked all the family to pray over him. Each of them laid their hands on Cheeseburger as his mother prayed. And did she pray – continuously for the next nine hours.

She prayed continuously for nine hours

The next day they returned to the Emergency Department for follow-up. The eye had healed.

———

Since he was a young child, Bruce has had the ability to predict when someone was getting ready to die. It began with his young friend Tom. He told his mother Tom was going to die. Disgustingly she asked, "Now how do you know that?!"

Despite her disbelief, for the next several days Bruce repeated that Tom was going to die. Tom in fact was healthy.

Soon afterwards, Tom became ill and entered the hospital. He never left. He died exactly two weeks after Bruce had first told his mother.

———

As an older child 50 years ago, Bruce lived in Smithtown, near Paris at a railroad crossing. One extended family, the Walden's, had several family houses there. In the Walden houses, there was always one room that no one was allowed in. Something secret happened behind those doors.

The oldest member, Ms. Walden, was in her 90s. Bruce was playing with about seven other boys when they saw her on a bluff not far away. All of the children rushed towards Ms. Walden with plans to tease her.

When she saw them coming, she pressed a finger on her nose and literally disappeared. There was no place she could have gone. They did not see her anywhere.

She pressed a finger on her nose and literally disappeared

The boys ran away in every direction! Bruce went home and hid under a chair. Many of those boys, to this day, refuse to talk about what happened.

As a child, Bruce was able to see people "that were not there." Sometimes he felt their presence. This typically was at dawn or dusk. They were nearly always friendly. Several he got to know quite well, including one he knew as Jim. Bruce's sense was they were there to help. Sometimes they would call him to come out of body to visit with them. At one point he in "real life" met a man who said, "I know you. We met out of body."

Only once did Bruce visit a house that had "unfriendlies." They chased him right out.

Bruce was always frightened about leaving his body. He worried when it happened if he was dying. Would he be able to get back into his body? He also worried other entities might get into his body.

Would he be able to get back in his body?

Bruce found it easy to leave the body, but a struggle to get back in. He both left and reentered his body through his feet.

In his early years, Bruce lived in a tiny community on the back of a historic Kentucky farm. One night his Grandmother Helen got up in the middle of the night. Very deliberately, she walked outside.

In Kentucky, there are "sinkholes" that form associated with the limestone formations in the ground. A sinkhole was near the house. It had suddenly gotten much larger, revealing caves.

Grandmother Helen walked down, with a rope wrapped around her. The rope extended from the top of the sinkhole to the entrance of one cave. Grandmother Helen spoke with someone who was in the cave. Bruce's mother Serena was at the top of the sinkhole watching and wondering.

The healer from the sinkhole caves

Serena's sister Betsy was crippled and could not walk. Whoever was in the cave gave his Grandmother advice on how to heal Betsy. Grandmother Helen was told to take the leftover table scraps of fruit and vegetables, put them in the dishwater and bathe this solution over Bruce's crippled aunt.

The next morning, the sinkhole had shifted. The cave entrances no longer were there. In time, Bruce's Aunt Betsy, though not perfectly, was able to walk again.

———

Bruce knew about God since six years old, but accepted him into his life at 12. He has been spiritual ever since.

Bruce was asked when to try to convert negative energy people. "Avoid evil people. Let God deal with them. But those who are weak and in need – those are the ones to focus on."

God knows about our problems, Bruce says, so do not pray about them. Instead, focus on praise and intention.

Once his car broke down with a water tank on the back. Bruce praised God for preventing it from happening on his steep driveway.

The Most Near-Deaths Ever?

GINNY has had an incredible eight near-death experiences, the most of anyone known! Her encounter with 12 robed beings. KENNA "channels," frustrated Jesus and experienced a Good Samaritan healing.

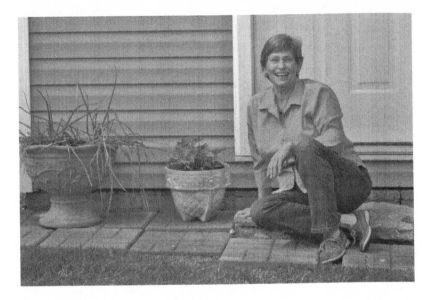

A sick feeling came over Ginny while teaching. 911 was called. At the emergency department, Ginny was told she had acid reflux. Two weeks later, Ginny heard a TV guest discuss his heart transplant. The guest kept repeating, "Do not get a heart transplant." Though she was by herself, Ginny said out loud: "I declare - no heart transplant!"

A week later, Ginny felt like she had been hit by a lightning bolt. A voice said, "Go to the emergency room now." It was the same voice she had heard after a horrible car accident 20 years earlier. She had not listened then. She did now.

When Ginny saw the look on the receptionist's face, she knew something was very wrong. The liquid for acid reflux that had worked three weeks earlier this time came up, hitting the opposite wall.

Then slow motion. Ginny could see everything. Fear blanketed the doctor and nurses faces. She heard a very calming voice say, "Be still." Then…complete peace. Though told she was stable enough for transport to Lexington, Ginny heard an EMT say, "She is not going to make it." She remembered thinking, "You should not say those things. Patients just might believe it." Later she realized no words had been spoken. She had read his thoughts.

During transport, Ginny found herself following the ambulance. It dawned on her. She was both inside *and* outside the ambulance.

Ginny rose. She was in a room with 12 robed beings of light. Through the glass walls, she saw planets throughout the universe.

She was with 12 robed beings of light

They used no words in talking, just images and feelings. This was different from school. This was like a Big School of Truth. Knowledge was being taught, but simultaneously with love.

Though sitting in a chair, Ginny could not see it. She could feel her hands and feet, but not see them with her earthly eyes but through her soul's eyes. As the council of 12 spoke, she understood everything.

On awakening, Ginny was told she needed a heart transplant to survive. She refused. She survived. In fact, she is fine.

* * * * *

Kenna was getting vertigo. Her doctor said it was not serious. But she heard an inner voice. It said she had to get outside. She ignored it.

The vertigo worsened. Kenna called her doctor who again reassured her. The voice again said, "Get out of the house," but she stayed in bed. When expressing concern to her husband, he encouraged her to rest more. She continued disregarding the voice.

Kenna continued to worsen. Her consciousness began to fade. She called her doctor, but he was reticent. Kenna recoiled. "I'm not asking! I'm insisting I be admitted to the hospital!" He agreed. But by now Kenna was extremely ill.

That night her family got ill and was hospitalized. A bat's nest had clogged the chimney triggering carbon monoxide poisoning.

Jesus appeared to Kenna, hands on his hips: "I told you to get out!"

Jesus: "I told you to get out!"

———

Kenna took her best friend Kim to a Waylon Jennings concert. The concert had barely started when Kenna saw flashes of blue light. She was being called to do healing. "Kim, we have to leave immediately!" All the way to the car, Kim fussed and fumed.

As they crossed the viaduct next to Rupp Arena, something appeared on the road ahead. Slowing down, they saw two people arguing. A man lay at their feet on the street. Blood poured from his head.

Kenna rushed from her car. She told the quarrelers to leave now! Kenna put her hands above the man's head. "I saw a river of water flowing from his head, running down the street."

The ambulance arrived and emergency medical technicians jumped to help. Kenna was firm. "Stay away." They complied.

With Kenna's treatment, the water reversed. She saw it flow back into his head. Intuitive friends interpreted this as his spirit "bleeding."

His spirit was bleeding from his head

When Kenna was through, there was no evidence of bleeding. Not wanting attention, Kenna and stunned Kim hurriedly left. The next day, the paper queried, "Who was this healing Good Samaritan?"

The Most Vivid Description of Heaven

BEVERLY's encounters with Jesus, Moses and Joseph, a guardian angel, a demon, life-saving intuition and scintillating near-death from an earthly saint

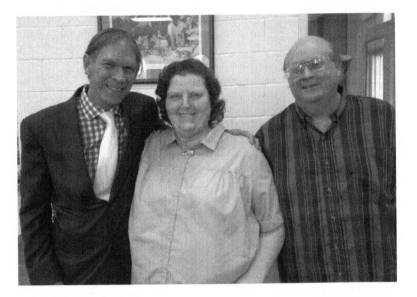

"I was run over by a tractor at eight years old. At the hospital, they found I had a broken back and a compound upper leg fracture. I was hurting so badly. Being a child, they were afraid to give me too much pain medicine. Mom and I prayed that Jesus would take my pain.

Jesus stood at the foot of my bed and took away my pain. I asked Momma who that was, but she could not see him. And he smiled. I did see his face.

Jesus is beautiful. He has dark skin and is strong, not at all wimpy, because he is a carpenter. He has good-sized hands, and took my whole foot in his hand." Beverly's eyes moistened as she described him."

A description of Jesus

———

"My guardian angel is as tall as this room. His bicep muscles and his thighs are a foot wide. You don't want to mess with him. He has been at the foot of my bed. He stands guard 24/7. I encounter him especially when I am ill or frightened. He takes away all of my fear."

———

"In the middle of the night, an angel woke me. I nearly bounced a foot off the bed! The angel said, 'Pray now!' I woke up my husband Johnny and told him we had to pray.

It turned out that exactly at the time the angel woke me, my brother had been in a terrible car accident. It had almost killed him."

———

"Dad died in a room at the old Lexington Veterans hospital. Mother, two sisters, two brothers and two friends were there. They were at the foot of the bed praying, except Mom was holding one hand, Sarah the other and I was at his elbow praying.

I prayed fervently. I wanted evidence Daddy was going to heaven. When he was young he had smoked, cussed and drank. He had quit drinking, but he did not stop cigarettes until forced to at the hospital. Daddy, though, had given his life to the Lord 10 years earlier.

We saw him take his last breath. Mom started crying. The room filled with angels. The tallest had his head bowed down because the room was not tall enough. The angels stood wingtip to wingtip all the way around the room. Another row of angels – shorter, 10 feet tall – were also wingtip to wingtip all the way around.

The room filled with angels

Then there was a row of people in white robes. I took that to be the

24 elders that are seated at God's throne.

Jesus descended down. He stood at the middle of Dad's tummy.
There was a robe over Jesus face, but you could see the nail scars in
both wrists.

Dad's spirit had the biggest most beautiful grin. Mom begged Dad
not to leave. He petted her hand and went back to Jesus. The clouds
rolled back, and they ascended toward heaven. The clouds then
reconnected and the top came back on the hospital.

A family member asked, 'Why didn't I see?' 'Because you did not
ask God to see.' Betty saw two angels, Sara saw one."

———

"I have awakened from a sound sleep speaking in tongues. One
language was Spanish. Another I think is American Indian, but I do
not know which tribe. This has happened hundreds of times."

———

"After Daddy died, Mom had to go to the hospital. She was very
sick. Daddy came to visit her there. My sisters Sara and Betty also
saw him and heard him. I think he came to get her. I told God I could
not live without my Momma. Betty agreed with me.

Daddy was not a ghost, but not a human either. You could tell all his
features, but he did not have skin and bones. He was whitish, but not
all white. His colors were inexplicable. Daddy seemed to have the
ability to see Mom. He left instantaneously.

We were all in the waiting room. Daddy came out to us. He talked to
us. My sisters about had a heart attack!

After his death, Daddy talked to us

'Did you see Dad? Did you hear that?'

Momma, though very sick, turned around. She was able to go

home."

———

"When there is something that goes really badly in Afghanistan, North or South Korea, or wherever American soldiers are stationed, I will be awakened in the night by an angel. I am shown a face. The angel asks me to pray. I will pray.

Usually it is my guardian angel that awakens me, but I have seen Gabriel, too. Gabriel awoke me with a trumpet call, just enough to wake me up.

Gabriel woke me with his trumpet

When growing up, beginning when I was six years old, Daddy told me to pray for the troops. My brother Jack was in the Korean conflict. Jack hit a bump in the road. There was a blast through the back of his seat. If he had not hit that bump, he would have been killed."

———

"Once I had the sudden awareness that something dangerous was wrong with Daddy. I heard him call my name. I loaded my kids in the car and took off to help him. We drove 45 miles to the family farm. When we arrived at his house, Mom was surprised we were there. I left the kids at the house with Mom. Driving to the back of the farm, I found Daddy. He had been run over by the tractor. If we had not found him, he might have died.

That has happened other times. While it has happened with others, it usually is family members."

———

Beverly one Saturday morning developed severe life-threatening symptoms. I was phoned at home to come immediately. I lived on the other side of our small town, just minutes away.

"I was having chest pain, shortness of breath and could not talk. My eyes were begging for help. The children went for Bill Mullins, an EMT up the street. Bill didn't touch me, backed into a corner and began praying. Bill had called the ambulance. Johnny had called you. I was breathing less and less deeply, more and more slowly. Why isn't anyone helping me?

All at once, it got dark. I saw the top of the house lift off.

"I saw the top of the house lift off"

I could see from where I was the ambulance on the railroad tracks a half-mile away. I could hear the ambulance driver and his partner talking about some lady on Second Street having chest pain. I saw the ambulance come down the street and turn in. I saw neighbors outside. I could hear their conversations. I knew what everyone was saying.

You came in. Johnny shared that I could not breathe. I could not fathom seeing all that. You asked me what was happening.

Everything went black. Over my head was a speck of light. Wonder what that is? Instantaneously, I was in heaven.

Jesus met me at the pearly gate. I know it was Jesus because the nail scar was in his wrists. It was not in his hands as some have said. I was not allowed to see his face. But I knew.

He took me through the gates and it was the most beautiful place. Flowers and grass and trees made music and sang. Angels were everywhere. They were singing. Their number was equal to the grains of sand.

"Flowers and grass and trees made music and sang"

There were no shadows under the trees. There was no darkness in heaven at all. Colors were so vibrant and bright. There is nothing on earth that compares.

I was with Jesus. At a certain point he said, 'They are praying for you and you have to go back, because I have to answer their prayers. You have to go back. I have work for you to do.'

I felt like I was falling really fast onto the couch. I had been given mouth-to-mouth resuscitation.

It was fantastic! I could hear God's booming voice. He was speaking to the angels because I could not make out what he said. God was in the background, but I only got just inside the gates.

It was a big pearly gate, mother of Pearl was what I saw. It was much more beautiful there than here. I walked on a street and could look down and see through it. It was as clear as crystal.

When I entered the gate, I saw earth. It looked like the end of a finger. It was blue as a marble.

I saw my mother and father, my grandmother and grandfather and my nephew Timmy Midkiff who died when he was 13. I saw others who I could not put a name to.

I saw Moses and Joseph because I asked to see them. I asked to see Jesus' face. He said no, not yet, but it would not be long.

"I saw Moses and Joseph"

Joseph was 5'6" and had a dark complexion. His eyes were almost black. He wore a turban on his head. He wore his coat of many colors. The colors almost jumped out at you.

There are animals in heaven – I saw horses, sheep, goats. That was as far back as I got. It resembled earth with hills, valleys and streams. The stream was small, but so blue. There was no air pollution.

I cried when Jesus said I had to come home. I said OK when he explained. I no longer fear death."

"I cried when Jesus said I had to come home"

Stories from My Travels

In the Business World from Boston to Chicago to Louisville, I finished presentations with my patient's spiritual experiences, generating excitement and positive energy. Even Mayo Clinic has a spiritual story.

Mother Mary's Embrace

Growing up, Tina's grandmother and grandfather took her to church.

When older, her grandmother used to say, "Put your problems in God's hands." "God gave me my own hands!" she would retort.

For three years after marriage, Tina was unable to get pregnant. She had stopped attending church. Finally she went. The next month she was pregnant – with twins.

A year later, a birthmark on the back of one twin, Lauren, signaled spinal deformity. The spinal cord was being dangerously stretched. Lauren required surgery.

In route to the hospital, Tina prayed to Mother Mary, who also had to worry about her son. "Give my daughter and I strength to handle the outcome, whatever that may be."

Suddenly, she felt an unmistakable, invisible embrace. Tina relaxed into a complete peace.

The surgery was high risk. But Lauren sailed through beautifully.

Ten years later, it was Tina's twin son Lyle. His surgery was urgent.

Once again she prayed to Mary. Again, Tina felt a full motherly embrace.

Immediately before surgery, she heard a voice: "He will be OK."

Lyle did beautifully.

* * * * *

After giving a business presentation that concluded with patient spiritual experiences, Lee Ann approached me. "Thank you for your comments."

Two years earlier, she had been sexually assaulted. It had been too much. Lee Ann's spirit left her body while this was happening. She observed herself successfully fend off the assaulter.

Later she heard the news. Her assaulter was being tried for the murder of *three* other women.

* * * * *

Though exceptionally bright, Henry had always had to deal with chronic depression. Medication only seemed to make things worse. When life started separating at the seams, Henry came to a decision.

He towered at the edge and then jumped from a seven-story building.

Near the bottom his forehead struck a telephone wire. His body flipped. Henry landed on his feet.

After a seven-story jump, he landed on his feet

He knew then there was a higher power. It was not his time. He was here for a purpose, and it was time to find out what that was.

At Mayo Clinic – Heavenly Chimes

In October of 2014, I presented at Mayo Clinic. It is a tremendous facility with immaculate grounds. Through the guidance of Brent Bauer, M.D., they are beginning to crack open their incredible potential through integrative health approaches. This story is from an employee assisting the presentation.

Shawn, a woman in her 50s, had a blissful near-death experience the year before. When sitting at home with her husband, he spoke loudly to her, "Did you hear that?"

No, Shawn had not heard anything.

He had heard chimes and voices speaking to him. He ran up right next to her and yelled, "Do you here THAT?"

She had not heard a thing.

Intuition acquired following her near-death experience taught her this could be an indication. They were coming to prepare him.

Thirty minutes later, he suddenly died.

A Solution to ALS?

Two reversals. GOD had a hand in both.

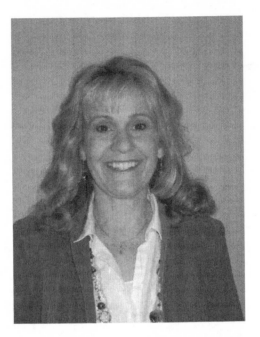

When Sue was 19, her family traveled to Acapulco. Jumping in the ocean, she had wandered a little far out. Suddenly, a rip tide carried her out to sea.

Sue struggled, but made no headway as the minutes passed away. No one seemed to notice. Exhausted, everything went black.

Then a voice. "Grab the rope!" But no one was there. Sue knew nothing of a rope. But what if there was? She thrashed her arms.

Then she felt it, the rough fiber against her hand. She grabbed with all her might. Somehow she pulled herself to shore.

Her family and others were aghast. She had been given up for dead.

She had been given up for dead

Despite this experience and exposure to church, Sue was not particularly religious. When 21, she was carousing with other inebriated young adults.

Sue was sitting shotgun when her friend carelessly pulled out in front of a car. Suddenly, she was face-to-face with a head on collision. Sue was terrified. On her right, she heard a voice: "Sue you will be alright."

She passed out. Then awoke in the emergency room intact.

Sue had it rough growing up in Jersey. Her father had been a successful, well-recognized TV businessman. At home, though, he had been abusive in many ways. While the family income was high, Sue would often go hungry.

Those experiences took a toll. Sue was anxious, obsessive and depressed. Powerful drugs were started for symptom control.

In a crowning blow, she was diagnosed in 1999 at 30 with amyotrophic lateral sclerosis (ALS, Lou Gehrig's Disease).

She was sensitive to loud noises and bright lights. Daily she struggled for energy. Muscles and joints ached. Eyes twitched. A mild tremor set in. Odd sensations came and went. Her heart would beat erratically. Progressively, she weakened. Her life was painfully fading.

But Sue was not a quitter; she had fought too many Jersey battles. For four years, every free moment was spent researching. She learned how toxic those drugs were. She was living in a cloud. It became brazenly clear. Sue had to get off those terrible drugs. From her reading, Sue learned to detoxify. Finally, she was "drug-free."

Her uncle, a minister, offered comfort and guidance. Nightly for an hour, she read scripture. It soon became obvious. Jesus wanted her to forgive her father. She could never truly heal until she had closed that hurt. Sue prayed, and then prayed more.

Jesus: Forgive your abusive father

Without giving details, Sue had a profound spiritual experience. It was the hope, the reassurance she had prayed for. Sue was given a promise. She would be healed.

Sue waited for instant resolution. It did not come. Instead, instant challenge. Her marriages had been a disaster. Now her second husband was announcing his departure.

Sue struggled. But now with a newfound, incredible energy.

Two months later, it was clear. All neurologic symptoms of ALS had faded away. She was going to survive...even thrive!

Sue recognized the special chance she had been given. Bound and determined, she would witness this gift! It was imperative to share her now extensive knowledge with others.

More years of study were rewarded with a naturopath degree. She learned most amazingly nearly all ALS was end-stage Lyme disease.

Most ALS is end-stage Lyme

Sue is a major intellectual and spiritual resource. Beyond three Amish communities in the states, her clientele extends across oceans from New Zealand to Saudi Arabia. Lyme is sexually transmissible. It is passed to children during pregnancy. All six of hers have Lyme, but her expertise keeps them well.

Last year, Sue invited her father and stepmother to come for a visit. They attended church together. Her dad committed his life to Christ.

Upon learning most ALS was Lyme, I became quite excited. Mike had been under my treatment for ALS the previous four months. While a nutritional and supplement program always helps, he was slowly weakening. Sensitive testing confirmed Lyme issues. This suddenly raised the prospect of reversal. Maximum intravenous antibiotic, plus two oral ones should give the answer.

Given in pulse fashion as recommended by Lyme experts, the first three days of each treatment Mike improved. On the fourth day, he had setbacks. Low-level laser therapy helped. Months later, Sue warned me of the crash in ALS after major antibiotic therapy.

After a month of stability, he began to sink. Collarbones and ribs protruded from sagging, wasting skin. Mike struggled to breath. In what surely was a death sentence, he developed pneumonia.

At the hospital, he was treated aggressively. Air hunger and low oxygen led to a tracheotomy and artificial ventilation. Doctors and nurses struggled to keep him alive. Many churches prayed for him.

But Mike was OK. He was in heaven "with Charlie." On horseback, Charlie joined farmer Mike in a beautiful place with waterfalls. Finally Charlie said, "You know Mike it is not your time yet. There are two or three other souls you need to save."

In heaven with Charlie on a horse

After five lost weeks, Mike began improving quickly. Defying the expected month-long hospital recovery, Mike was home in two weeks.

At home, Mike's strengthening continued. At his last visit with his ALS doctor, the doctor was so shocked that he brought in a colleague to see him. "Whatever you are doing, keep doing it!"

Mike is back on supplements and his laser treatments. Incredibly, he is now walking 15 feet on his own power for the first time in a year.

He walked 15 feet for the first time in a year

Sue has shared with me her successful strategy. So many of her clients get better. After struggling four years to get a handle on Lyme, we are excited at what Sue's new approach will accomplish in Midway.

Mike, a gentle, loving soul, offers living testimony to those of us in the healing profession and to God. Our office will do everything we can to help Mike save those two or three souls.

An Archangel, Demons and a Time Traveler

Flying to Minneapolis led to discovery of rich stories. Betty was spiritually gifted to deal with immense challenges. Karen and Armand are bright young adults. Heather takes psychiatry to a whole new spiritual level. It was only due to one of "God's coincidences" that these stories were to be shared with me for this book.

My plane out of Philadelphia was stuck on the tarmac, taking over an hour to get in the air. Chicago I knew would be an incredibly close air connection. I prayed to God. "Thy will be done. If I am to make this connection, so be it. But if I miss it, I recognize it as your plan."

The connecting gate was nearby. But when I arrived, it had closed. Seeing the plane still connected, I banged on the gate door. But the attendant who came refused to allow me on the plane.

A woman, who was also late, was sobbing. So much needed to be done that weekend! On the next plane out to Minneapolis, we ended up next to each other in the last row. It turned out to be Beth, one of the most incredible persons I have ever met.

Karen and Armand, the two check-in persons at my Minneapolis hotel, I never would have met if I had arrived on the earlier plane. All of these fascinating stories I would have missed had I made the connection!

* * * * *

Beth Baeur knew Christ beginning at four when at Sunday school; she realized, "Oh, that's the missing piece." Ever since, Beth has been aware of spiritual gifts. She began to see auras and have dreams that would come true on a regular basis. She would know things before they would happen. Beth can scan the body, identify problem areas, and then heal them. Beth can even diagnose and heal over the phone. Jesus tells her if she can heal someone or not.

With Jesus' OK, she can scan the body, diagnose and heal

Though her life has been especially challenging, never in her life has Beth been upset or angry with God. Her gifts may have been preparation for these challenges. Specifically two sons have muscle anomalies requiring power chairs, tracheotomies, ventilators and feeding tubes. Both are spiritual, especially Alex, her oldest.

Beth's second son, Levi, had a near-death experience when he was only three months old. His feeding tube migrated into, and perforated, his intestines, making him very ill. Beth knew he was sick, but doctors dismissed it. She insisted he stay in the hospital. The next morning it was clear how ill he was. They had to repair his intestines. He died four different times in a two-week period. The only thing that would bring him back was Beth talking to him and touching him. He was in the ICU for two months. The day he went home, the doctor hugged Beth and told her that Levi was a miracle.

"Ever since when Levi touches you, it feels like you are being touched by something heavenly, like an angel. It is an unreal feeling."

Alex has had four near-death experiences. One was after a surgical attempt to put a rod in his back for his severe scoliosis. Beth intuited the rod mistakenly went into his lung. Doctors dismissed it as pleural fluid but she knew the truth. Because they refused to acknowledge it, she had him transferred.

Alex's lung re-expanded. The chest tube was to be removed, but Beth had a premonition this would kill him. She refused the procedure.

A second surgery was required to remove the lung clot caused by the rod damage. A large blood clot was keeping the ripped lungs held together as the rod perforated his lung, not just the lung sac. The surgeon later told Beth she was 100 percent right; had they removed the chest tube in his room, he would have died instantly.

For no logical reason, the anesthesiologist felt compelled to have blood on hand. During the surgery Alex lost seven of the eight units of blood normally in the body. If blood had not been instantly ready, Beth was told, her son would have died from blood loss.

Beth once had a premonition that with one son on a stair lift platform leading up from the basement, the lift would collapse. It would kill the other son down below.

Beth ignored the premonition. After escorting Alex on to the stair lift, Beth began to pray that her premonition wouldn't happen. Halfway up, she saw Levi drive onto the bottom of the stairs. Frantically she yelled, "Get out of the way!" He drove off as the lift collapsed. Beth grasped Alex's chair so that he wouldn't plunge down the stairs. The tumbling 450-pound chair would have crushed Levi. Had Beth not acted quickly Levi would have died and probably Alex too.

A premonition saves both sons

Beth realized shortly after marriage she could act on premonitions to prevent them. She foresaw that on a trip to visit her Grandmother their car would have a flat tire and their house would be robbed.

The car had a flat and on return home, their house had been robbed.

Both sons are in religious colleges. Alex while there has had to deal with demons. He would get lower respiratory infections. Beth could intuit from a long distance he had a demon in his lungs. While he was ill, Beth visited every day to do healing. One day as Beth entered his room, she immediately heard him wheezing. As she began to work on Alex, she could feel the demon behind him. As he had a new nurse who she didn't want to scare, Beth whispered the words to cast the demon away. Instantly, Alex stopped wheezing. His nurse exclaimed, "That's incredible!" Beth figured the nurse assumed she had healed him. Correcting her might frighten her. Alex exclaimed, "I feel awesome!" and immediately started homework. Before this, Alex had been tired and had difficulty thinking.

On another day a different nurse saw things moving around the room. Beth used an exorcism book to get the devil out. That same day, a friend trying to get into the son's room heard steps and movement in the room but no one was in the room. It took several attempts to drive the demons away.

Beth has felt demons when doing her energy work. She can exorcise them using a specific book and words that God has given her to say.

Beth recognizes and exorcises demons

Once as she was exorcising, a deep raspy voice from a frail older woman asked, "What are you doing? Are you sure you know what you are doing? This doesn't feel right!" The demon then left.

She finds those who use drugs, including marijuana, always have demons. Once demons are dealt with, drug craving immediately resolves.

Beth once brought a bottle of water from the river of Jordan to Alex. Before knowing it was special, Alex as he held it remarked, "Wow, Mom, this really has a lot of love and energy!"

Beth also has the vision of arrows entering her left shoulder. She recognizes this comes from a previous life. Someone had been with Beth in her past life that is now in her current life. This person vividly remembers details of their past lives together.

* * * * *

She was tired of it all. Karen had decided she would end her life.

Grouped before her was an assortment of pills that she felt would work.

As she lay in bed, Karen noticed something odd reflecting off of the TV. She looked closer. There was much movement in the reflection. A fleeting pointed tail here, a pair of horns there. Frighteningly evil faces were there for an instant, then back out of view.

She counted. Reflecting from her front door onto the TV, there were four of them. Four devils. They were waiting impatiently. They were waiting for her. If there is hell, there must be heaven. And if there is heaven, there is a reason to live. Karen threw away her pills.

Four devils awaited her suicide

In church, and to anyone who will listen, she testifies about what she saw. This transformed her life. Karen is now a bright, delightful, upbeat and immaculately dressed young woman. She appreciates and loves her life. Karen is a disciple for her Christ.

* * * * *

Armand and a friend were awakened in the middle of the night. A guy with a T-shirt on his head walked in to their bedroom. His clothes were ragged. He had a jean jacket. Parchment was around his lower chest with three odd symbols. He was a real enigma.

Parchment and three odd symbols

The visitor went to the bookshelf and pulled down a book. It instantly opened to a section on the origin of man, beginning as apes in Africa.

He was very knowledgeable, his accent unusual. The three talked well into the night. Earlier that day, the visitor had been to two lost cities overseas. But they were not the ones we are aware of today.

When Armand left the room for 10 seconds and returned, the visitor was gone. Armand's roommate witnessed, participated in and was awe-struck about what had transpired.

Earlier, he had been to two lost cities

* * * * *

For decades, Heather had explored spiritual connections. As a holistic psychiatrist from Rhode Island, she had learned much about "the other side."

As a client, Heather knew Salina well. They had been close friends for many years.

Now though, Salina was in an intensive care unit comatose.

Heather put her hand over Salina's heart. A journey began.

Salina escorted her up into her near-death experience. For an hour, Heather was able to experience what heaven was like.

Heather escorted her up into her spiritual near-death experience

———

Heather had a patient, Cary, who attempted suicide. In the process, she went out of her body. What happened next was unusual.

Another spirit entered Cary's body and took charge. The voice was more bass. The "new" Cary was apathetic in her actions.

Heather, determining what had happened, came up with a plan. It would take much assistance, but she felt it could work.

She called upon Archangel Michael. Heather's dead father was also summoned to help this thieving spirit to transition to the other side.

A spirit snatches her body. Archangel Michael to the rescue

Heather then asked the spirit in Cary's body if it could see the bright light. It responded, "Yes, so what?"

Heather could still detect a hang up. She got further heavenly assistance. Heather then told the spirit to go to the bright light. It did, leaving Cary's body.

Cary could then reenter her body. Her life was back!

Quantum Leap with the Most Incredible Story

Steve and Bill Harrison fulfill your author and media potential. GOD's pathway to the next level of achievement and eclipsing a business collapse!

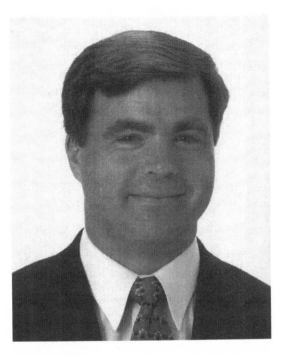

"'If you don't come back with at least twenty-thousand dollars next weekend, we're going to be out of business!'

When I heard my brother Bill say those words, I froze.

I was so afraid and unsure what to do that even though I was sitting in his office, I felt like I was in a prison cell with the walls and ceiling slowly collapsing all around me.

There was no way out.

As calmly as he could, Bill explained that our credit line was completely maxed out. We needed to make payroll, and we simply didn't have enough money.

That's why we needed $20,000 and we needed it fast. If we didn't have that money soon, we were going to have to lay everyone off.

We needed $20,000 and needed it fast

Bill and I had been business partners for fourteen wonderful years. Our company had helped launch such bestselling books as *Chicken Soup for the Soul, Men are From Mars Women are From Venus* and *Rich Dad Poor Dad*. We'd gone from working out of a modest two-bedroom apartment and had created a successful multi-million dollar company. Thousands of entrepreneurs, authors and speakers gave us credit for helping them market themselves effectively.

But right now, none of that mattered. In fact, it made me feel worse. If I was so good at sales and marketing, why was I about to go broke?

What was I going to say to the eight wonderful employees, whose families really depended on their incomes?

Our sales had taken a sharp downturn in the wake of the 9/11 tragedy. For several months, it seemed like no one was buying anything, but our fixed expenses kept draining our bank account.

Things just seemed to get worse and worse.

I'd go to the ATM machine to get cash for lunch, and it would simply show me two words: "Insufficient Funds."

When my wife said, 'I'm really worried. You're working day and night. I never see you. I can't put these bills off any longer? How are we going to pay them?' I started to cry.

When my wife asked, "How are we going to pay the bills?" I started to cry

During this time, I read an interview by a Christian author and former priest named Bennan Manning. He recommends that you pray by simply talking to God with your eyes wide-open as if he were sitting in a chair next to you. He even encourages you to pull up an actual chair! The most important thing is to be completely honest and then listen to what he might say.

One day, I was walking in a field near my office talking aloud to God in prayer. Suddenly, I started crying. In my anger and frustration, I yelled: 'God, why is this happening to ME!'

GOD, Why is this happening to me?

He didn't answer.

So brother suddenly told me we needed $20,000 in one weekend. I didn't know what I was going to do. Was God going to let me lose my business? Did he have something else planned for me?

I was scheduled to speak at a conference in California that weekend.

I'd been there several times before, but each time I would barely come back with enough money to pay my travel expenses.

How was I possibly going to go there this time and bring back $20,000?

I began to think about what if anything I could do to better serve the audience and what I might be able to offer them.

I'd never used PowerPoint before, but I went to the effort to create some slides. Then I flew to the conference in California determined to do my best.

Right before I went on, I experienced a lot of computer problems. It looked like I wasn't going to be able to use my PowerPoint at all.

I was sunk.

What was I going to say to my brother?

My heart was pounding in my chest.

I was terrified.

I could hear those words, 'If you don't bring in at least $20,000, we'll be out of business.'

But right before I went on I said to myself, 'Don't worry about any of that. Just love and serve the people in the audience.'

Just love and serve the people...

Suddenly, my PowerPoint was working. I spoke freely and passionately. In fact, it was going so well, I couldn't believe it was me actually speaking!

It felt like it was someone else, a newer, better version of me.

I shared specific ideas and strategies that entrepreneurs, experts and authors can use to get the word out about what they are doing.

The moment of truth came towards the end of the talk. I was allowed to give a brief commercial about my company's service and let people know about a special discount package I was offering at the conference. I handed out a yellow order form for anyone who was interested.

Before I finished speaking, a lady came walking down the aisle and handed me her order form! Then another person came and another! People were mobbing the stage to hand in their order forms before I'd even finished speaking!

People were mobbing the stage

I got so choked up I couldn't talk. In that very instant, I remembered a Bible story I'd learned long ago.

Jesus tells his disciples to put down their nets for a catch. They replied, 'Master, we've been fishing all night and haven't caught anything, but because you say so, we will let down the nets.' They then instantly catch so many fish their nets were literally breaking. When I saw all these people coming forward, I felt my nets bursting.

I didn't receive $20,000 that day.

I received $67,000.

When I called Bill on the phone and shared with him the amount of money that had come in, he said, 'You did what?'

He couldn't believe it. He was thrilled and relieved all at once.

But I actually received much more than money that day. I received a new calling on my life.

God used that experience to reinvent my business and reinvent me.

GOD used that experience to reinvent my business and me

I ultimately became a much more successful speaker, coach and consultant.

Today, entrepreneurs, authors, and speakers fly to me from around the world to participate in my trainings, seminars and coaching programs. I'm able to share with them the secrets for shaping and sharing their message for maximum impact and income.

And I know from experience that no matter what kind of difficulties

I experience , God is 'the God who sees me' (Genesis 16:13)."

For free training on how to become a more successful author, speaker or entrepreneur, go to www.steveharrison.com or www.bestsellerblueprint.com

* * * * *

Vivacious, attractive Claire was impressively full of spiritual energy as she made her presentation. Afterwards, in complementing her ideas, Claire shared that her life had made a dramatic turn. Six months earlier, she had a long fall while hiking, landing forcefully on her head. While steadily recovering, she is not all the way back.

This was astounding. Her presentation had been sterling. How good would she be when "all the way back?"

Of more surprise, she was grateful for the experience. She had been in an affair. Her life was continually contorted to maintain secrecy to fulfill each other's boundless needs. She bounced from one stressful moment to the next.

While falling, she had a near-death experience. God revealed to her fully how her life was destroying herself and others. Afterwards, she immediately began a new life. With a close college friend, she has started a new, promising business venture.

GOD revealed how she was destroying herself and others

* * * * *

Paul Walker, from the hit series *Fast and Furious*, had died in a car accident. Shula had heard of Paul, but had never met him. But weeks after his death, she suddenly was overcome by his presence. Shula, a humble, shy woman, had been gifted with spiritual intuitiveness. Never had she experienced the presence of anyone so powerfully.

Paul was distraught. When he visited his loved ones and his son, they did not respond. It was as if he was not there. Even at work, he had difficulty getting anyone to listen.

Shula understood. He was challenged transitioning to the other side. She knew an intuitive that could help.

Even stars need help transitioning

Two weeks later, Paul successfully transitioned. Shula still gets messages from Paul. But now they are messages of immense gratitude.

* * * * *

Anthony was always close to his father. Following his father's death, he visited his father's grave in Italy.

Normally graveyards in Italy are considered very scary places. But Anthony felt calm.

Then a wind pushed him away. He got the message, "Shush back home. You don't need to be here. Get on with your life!"

For two years after his father's death, Antony would dream about him.

One morning he awoke and couldn't move. Antony felt his father's embrace. He could feel him touch his cheek.

His father said, "Why do you worry about me? I am fine. Stop worrying!"

* * * * *

Roy Martina, M.D. and his wife Joy were highly successful holistic practitioners and trainers in Europe. One day they received a spiritual message to move to America. They suggested to God they were happy where they were or would, if he insisted on them changing location, prefer to move to a place by the beach. But God made it very clear to them that they needed to move to their specific sanctuary in the mountains. And so they followed suit and gave up everything they had in Europe to relocate to the US. They now live in Asheville, North Carolina and are blissfully happy there. They say this move was the best thing they could have done and are amazed at how precise God was in his guidance.

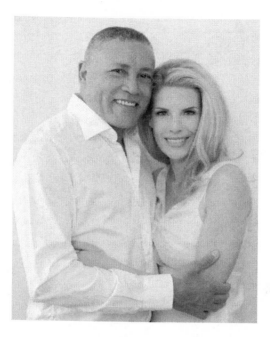

At GOD's insistence, they gave up everything in Europe for America

Joy and Roy are both hypnotists and trained in remote viewing. Joy is a highly effective channeler and together they have trained hundreds of people to do the same and become their own oracles. Joy and Roy work as a team, so when Joy channels, Roy is excellent in asking the questions that lead to very insightful conversations with the spirit world and astonishingly accurate and helpful answers. In their sessions, they ask who is best to deal with the challenge or issue at hand. Roy suggests that while Jesus is good to channel for many things, it is better to call on practical spirits for specific problems.

Insightful conversations with the spirit world through channeling

* * * * *

One saving grace is that Shari had a good friend at work, Christopher. The two had promised that whoever died first would come back and tell the other what it was like. Unexpectedly, Christopher died weeks later.

Shari now hosts a TV show. As a special guest, she had Theresa, a psychic "medium." In the middle of the show, Theresa's train of thought was suddenly interrupted. The medium shared a spirit was trying to contact Shari.

The spirit stated his date of birth as the date of Christopher's death, typical of Christopher's quirky humor. His personality was the same, as were Theresa's description of his height and other characteristics.

Finally, the spirit shared two things that only Christopher and Shari knew. Christopher indeed was visiting. He had kept his promise.

Christopher kept his promise to visit from the other side

* * * * *

Three near-death experiences had transformed John into a spiritual man. At four a.m., he was aroused from his slumber. Intuitively he was told, "Personally deliver a message to your chiropractor."

Ray Drury, D.C.'s office was three hours away. But John knew despite his old age that it was imperative he make the trip. Upon arriving, he immediately summoned Ray who he knew well. Dr. Drury was very surprised to see John. He knew John was not on the schedule. Ray also knew that it was a long trip for the old man.

John was direct with Dr. Drury. "God told me that there is an employee working for you whose name is Butler. It is Butler's intention to do you harm. He told me I must warn you immediately."

GOD told him to drive three hours to rescue his chiropractor from an evil employee

John delivered this message never having met Butler. In fact, he had never heard Butler's name.

Three months earlier, Dr. Drury hired Butler to manage Shirley and Cassandra, two recently hired employees. Taking charge immediately, Butler told the other two not to ever say anything critical to the boss about him. If they disobeyed his orders, they would be fired!

Butler's actions, however, seemed outlandish to the two women. It was clear Butler had his own agenda. That agenda had nothing to do with improving patient care or office profitability.

One day it became so bad that Shirley knew she had to challenge Butler. She was not expecting what happened next. Butler's eyes became fiery. His face turned red. She watched in terror as it became distorted, misshapen.

She watched in terror as his face became distorted, misshapen

Dr. Drury knew John's spirituality. He greatly respected him as both a patient and a dear friend. After quickly interrogating Shirley and Cassandra, Dr. Drury fired Butler immediately.

* * * * *

"One morning I was in the shower in the front bathroom when a tidal wave of unconditional love filled the whole of my being. I was aware the body was crying and there was no distinction between myself and the shower water. Not only had the water become me and I the water, but in that moment I was everything. I was one with the Divine. There was no separation between who I was and the air, the room, the house, the whole of the universe. I was one with all that is. The True Self had completely annihilated the ego mind's elaborate construct of subject and object, of duality and separation.

I had the vague awareness that my body was still in existence, but I was totally detached from it other than to know that it too was only a tiny particle in the whole of the cosmos, in the mind of the Divine. I was a sublime, drunken puddle of unconditional love merged into God's grace. Unconditional love coursed through the Divine Mind, which had enveloped my mind where nothing else existed.

Everything finally disappeared into this love. I was not frightened because fear simply cannot exist in this state and I had already had similar experiences of being in this state of awe, oneness and love.

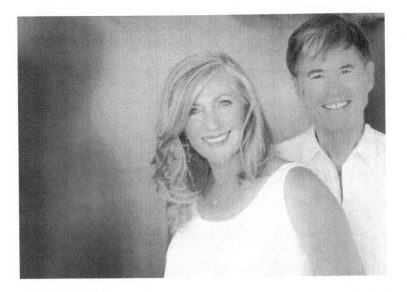

Somehow I had turned off the water and was stepping out of the shower when Daniel walked from his office at the other end of the house into the bathroom. Glowing with joy, he dropped to his knees, tears flowing, overwhelmed by the waves of energy filling the entire apartment emanating from the center of what used to be my being.

He wrapped his arms around my waist, and leaning his head into my wet stomach, he said, 'I just tracked down the source of the waves of energy that enveloped me in the most beautiful, unconditional love and total acceptance.'

We weren't drunk or on drugs, but we were both drunk and high in the real world of unconditional love where the heart sings with unbridled joy. In this world, forgiveness accomplishes the impossible; all life is one in all of its beauty and splendor. And this is who we all are; it is our true nature. When you reenter the real world of God, you are perfect beyond the ego mind's ability to comprehend.

You are perfect beyond the ego mind's ability to comprehend

When Buddha said, 'I am awake,' he meant he realized he was not merely a participant in the illusory world of the ego mind, but the creator of the entire illusion. This is from one who had become whole in his essence. He woke up to the truth that the world we live in is solely the creation of the ego mind running wild in its dreamlike state.

The love in the shower experience took us beyond the realm of our ego minds, and reality moved in on us. When it finally subsided, we were awake to the fact that if it is not divine love, then it is not real.

From the age of three, divine beings have been conversing with me and guiding my life on every level. As a four-year-old, I told my mother I was here to work for God because that is what I knew to be true from my beloved divine friends. Living in a state of enlightenment where you are aware you are not only connected to but one with all life means you are living the best version of you. Here is to us living the light and love that we are!"

From the age of three, divine beings have been conversing with me

Sandra and Daniel Biskind excerpts from their book *LOVE: Ignite The Secret To Your Success.*

* * * * *

At a Philadelphia restaurant before my Quantum Leap conference, I was anxious to meet others trying to further their career. Sitting by himself was Dr. Jay Roberts, a man who has changed my life.

Dr. Roberts has a pain clinic near Palm Springs, California. Growing up, Jay suffered major abuse from his war-hero father, Roy. His father wanted Jay to be tough. When Roy got drunk, he lashed Jay with a whip. He never showed love. He wanted a "tough" son.

Jay had an imaginary friend, Buddy. When Roy was getting ready to beat him, Jay would escape in his mind with Buddy. They would go to the playground or look for adventure. Buddy was always there and always had answers for Jay in his time of need.

When he turned 18, his father let him move to the Philippines in care of the Governor, a war buddy. Jay attended medical school there and did mission work when he had the opportunity. He was proud of being able to help. He witnessed healing from prayer – miraculous healing.

Jay experienced other miracles on these mission trips. Once he fell off a cliff. He landed 40 feet below, on the only bush that was nearby.

He landed 40 feet below, on the only bush that was nearby

At one point, in a remote area of the Philippines, he had barely escaped headhunters. During a revolution, he had precariously survived.

After an exemplary medical residency in America, Jay was very successful. He treated many movie stars. Jay treated pain without narcotics using safe, effective, non-addicting Thor low level lasers. He subsequently wrote the FDA manual on low-level laser therapy.

Then everything changed. He acquired an autoimmune illness very much like ALS. Jay's body began to deteriorate. He was slowly dying.

Jay's wife Beverly had a strong faith. She encouraged Jay to visit Lourdes, France. In Chicago, a priest, Father Rookey, gave Jay a prayer. "Read this prayer in all sincerity and you will be healed," Father Rookey promised. Included was a line about forgiveness.

Jay did not understand why he was dying. Where was God? When he was a child, he prayed to God to free him from the abuse. But God never did. Jay felt that God was not there.

He fervently petitioned God. "Give my illness to prisoners. They have done bad things. They are the ones who deserve this!"

Now death was nearing. God was nowhere to be found.

Jay lost use of his arms and legs. His doctors had lost hope. Hospice was consulted. Jay was weeks from death. He purchased his casket.

He purchased his casket

He pleaded with God. He had a rough life. Jay deserved a break.

After fighting hard to defeat his illness, after praying daily, Jay finally surrendered. "Thy will be done, not my will."

For the first time, he said Father Rookey's prayer with sincerity about forgiving his father. And he said the Lord's Prayer.

A white cloak passed over his head. He felt Jesus' presence. He experienced complete peace. Jay then drifted off to sleep. In the morning, miraculously, he hopped out of bed. His arms and legs worked fine. He could not believe it!

His neurologist was very excited. Even though it was excruciatingly painful, his doctor wanted a nerve biopsy for a case report in a major medical journal. Jay refused. The neurologist cursed.

Now along with his work at the pain clinic, he spends three days every month locked up with the most hardcore criminals. He was nearly killed once by new convicts who were not familiar with his work. But he successfully continues his work.

He spends three days a month locked up with the most hardcore criminals

Patients sometimes show up at his office with a single request – that he pray for them.

He has bought land in the Philippines where he will be building an orphanage for 100 children. A clinic will be set up nearby where he can do surgery and provide medical care.

Jay is a cheerful individual with a big smile. Without a doubt, he says, what was killing him was unforgiveness for his Dad. Jay's book, *Break The Chains*, made me cry and made me laugh – it is terrific!

* * * * *

Julie Renee Doering was born autistic, could not speak until she was five, was born with a tangled intestines and without some bones. "I have seven nieces and nephews that have some version of autism... Life was very, very challenging. I literally survived the atomic bomb testing as a child and went through 17 surgeries, multiple cancers, I died a couple of times and spent a year of my life in a wheelchair.

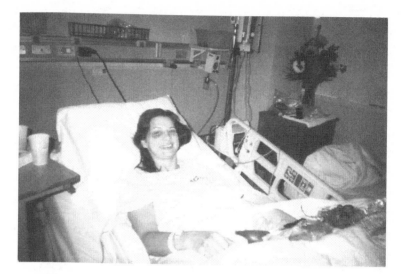

I discovered I had cancer when I was pregnant with my third child and was told I would probably not survive the pregnancy. But my doctors did not talk to me about abortion even though they thought it might be an option to save my life because they knew I was a woman of faith and would say no. Sure enough, being a woman of faith helped me survive. I prayed three hours a day for my baby and when he was born he was eight lbs. I was 104 pounds at that point, just skin and bones, but I had this big, fat, healthy baby and the power of prayer really worked."

Julie Renee had two spiritual near-death experiences, one most startling. "I had infection of my brain and heart, and I was shaking. When the angel came over me I was ice cold, I remember it very clearly. The angel looked male, but it was definitely the angel of death. 'OK, you can come with me.' 'Get thee behind me Satan, I am not going with thee. I know you are not Satan, you are the angel of death, but I am going nowhere with you. I am holding on to this body, I am not going with you, you cannot make me go.'

Born autistic, she did not speak until age five

Years later, having survived many traumas and many difficulties, I came to a point in my life where my kids were grown and I felt like I could not tolerate the pain any longer. I had told my oldest daughter, 'Honey just pull the plug if anything else happens, I am not going to fight this day, I cannot be in this pain anymore,' and she said to me, 'Mom, I do not want you to be in pain… I want you to feel better, I want you to live and I do not want you to die.'

I started thinking about that and that opened up a door for me. It was really remarkable. The door that it opened was I had really not put in my formula that I was to go beyond surviving, that I was going to get to 100 percent. The only thing I had ever really focused on was surviving. I did a great job of surviving, but I was in pain and difficulty and illness all the time. So I changed that request to, 'God heal me completely, God make me well or take me.' I really had felt like that up until that point I had been living in hell for many, many years and that I was now declaring that I was ready to live in the Garden of Eden no matter what.

Wheelchair-bound and suffering, she asked for the Garden of Eden

In that decision, I had earlier in my life gone to where Buddah was enlightened and I actually sat under the Bodhi tree, a distant grandchild of the original Bodhi tree that Buddah sat under in India. And I knew his story. He had been told he was the son of a wealthy king, and he would never have the possibility of being enlightened. Yet he went and sat under the tree and meditated for days on end, and he did become a wise, enlightened being. I had that same feeling that I needed to declare I deserved the Garden of Eden, that I deserved mastery and joy in the body, and that I deserved this incredible life, this opportunity of being in a human body.

I always felt like that I was here for a reason. I always felt this suffering…was for something. But I did not know what it was for. Going into the garden and declaring that opened up the door to my memories, and opened up the door to me becoming the person who I was meant to be. I went into my garden in prayer and meditation, and just like Buddah, I said, 'God, I am here and I am not leaving until I receive this kind of enlightenment, this experience of joy and power in the body.' And that is exactly what started happening the very first day." A blue glow emanated from her abdomen. "I began to watch cells regenerating in my body. It was an incredible experience. It was like looking at the face of God as I watched His master cells go to the perfected God state. And from there I continued to heal." Her intestinal tract and organs fully reshaped. Even her tonsils reappeared.

Julie Renee had been told she would never walk again. But though wheelchair-bound, she determinedly learned to walk with canes. Then the transformation: "I began to walk without canes. I had unbearable pain in my legs and (after two weeks)…all of a sudden I had no pain in my legs, and I could run and dance. You must understand that the person who was told that she would return to the wheelchair, that determination was keeping me out, after six months I was running 30 miles a week on a mountain and I was dancing on stage with a rock 'n roll band every week.

So these incredible things started happening and the doctors around me were saying, 'How are you doing this, what is going on with you?' And eventually a couple of the doctors convinced me to start teaching them. What that meant for me in the first six months of trying to teach doctors was I had to translate and create a language of how to describe what it was I saw, what it was I was working with, the quantum field, the cells and the DNA. So for a while I was in this kind of phase where I felt like I was translating a heavenly knowledge to an earthly language. I was defining, 'What am I doing? How is this working?'

Julie Renee's body regenerated

That was indeed my path…this is what I was meant to do, and that there was a purpose for all the suffering. The suffering made so much sense, it was meant to help humanity, it was meant to change the way we see our bodies and our lives.

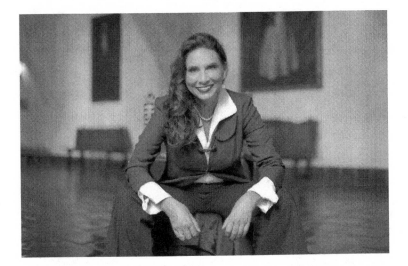

Had I not suffered as much as I did…had I not gone through the difficulties and the trials I would not have been believable to others, but having died, having had multiple cancers, having had all these terrible things happen to me and then being fully recovered, healed and 100 percent, I can really stand as an example for others who have suffered to say, 'We are powerful beyond measure, we are radiant beams of light, we come with an innate ability to heal.' Healing is natural…the quantum field is meant to regenerate and rejuvenate us for hundreds of years, and that maybe not in our lifetime, but certainly in the future people will go back to living hundreds of years.

I felt like what I was really to do was to show people how to regenerate the body, how to enjoy, how to celebrate every moment of every day, how to break the financial blocks, how to clear the entanglements with love, which are all wired into the blueprint. We come with this incredible system to help us heal in every way."

I first met Julie Renee at Quantum Leap in Philadelphia. Her health was exceptional. She spoke rapidly with clarity and purpose. There was no evidence that she had ever experienced ill health.

"I have worked with people in the Pentagon and the United Nations. I was offered a job for remote viewing, and I turned it down. I just morally could not. I felt like it was definitely not what I wanted to do. On the search and rescue, I had been asked many times to help with missing children and have been blessed to actually help restore some children just before death to where they were actually rescued and survived. But the last couple were very gruesome where the children were mutilated. I did not have the heart for it.

Her remote viewing saved children

From the time of childhood, I felt like I had to go to India. I finally got there at age 33, and when I arrived it was like everybody remembered me. I had been a teacher there a number of times, and people would bow down and kiss my feet everywhere I went. When I came to one guru, he said, 'Where have you been? I have been looking for my entire life for you. I have searched the whole globe and now I am an old man ready to die.' It was just this beautiful homecoming. India felt like home. Everybody remembered me. It was so sweet, and I knew that I was to get the work out in the West, but I also needed to have this experience of being home…being at ease and having that kind of love and reverence. Back then I needed that fortification. I needed that acknowledgement and that love to give me courage to go on. Even the men with the shotguns in the airport, they bowed down and touched my feet, everybody did, so for me it was like, 'OK, I'm supposed to be here.' Now I feel like I am working on my purpose….I just feel like everything has been divine flow, everything is going extremely well."

She was worshipped in India

At the time of her enlightenment, Julie Renee became aware of her previous lives. She learned she was from another planet and that this was her sixth life here. After this life, she is to return to that planet. "I feel when I accessed my memories that I was part of the human divine team. I came back and have done six lifetimes to help restore the knowledge that was built into us, that was wired into humanity. So I feel like I was part of that team that created that beautiful design. I know it sounds a little schizophrenic. I am a woman of faith and I was part of the design team, but somehow they really do make sense to me."

After this, her sixth life here, she will return to another realm

Julie Renee had communicated with the spirit of Gandhi at one point and interacted with Nelson Mandela in her mind's eye on the evening after he had died before she had heard the news. "I was hearing his speech, but it was coming in very personal, as if our thoughts were merging and he was giving me the blessing of his vision and inspiration. In the dark after a long time of being present to his essence, I wrote my impression of our commingling thoughts:

Nelson Mandela visits in transition

Who are you to play small? You, who would just survive, defer dreams and ignore the gifts and talents you were gifted? Having 'survived' the worst of human health challenges, even death itself, I ask you now if you can honestly say you are playing your life at 100 percent?

If the living of your life were measured like an Ivy League grading system, could you say in all aspects of your life, health, relationships and expression that you were indeed living to your full potential? Are you planning to get your work and mission into the world in this lifetime while you have momentum and ability to fulfill your vision?

You were born into this life charged with a mission and a purpose. Why are you holding back? Everything you need to fulfill your divine purpose is already within you. By holding back your light, your love, your vision, you deny all of us humans the deepest gifts of your essence.

I charge you to live life full; with a generosity and gratefulness to change heaven and earth for the betterment of all. Deny me not the privilege of your best 100 percent life. You are so much more than you have shared to this point. Isn't now the time to live 100 percent?"

Julie Renee's website is www.julierenee.com

Epilogue

This journey for me has been incredibly fulfilling. It has positively transformed my life. Do I have a "knowing" about Jesus and God? Yes. Have I witnessed God's impact on the world? Repeatedly. Are these stories for real? What you may not always appreciate as a reader is how sincerely and humbly these stories are shared. I can assure you these individuals are connected to God. And I can verify these stories fundamentally changed those that experienced them in a profoundly positive and life-altering way. The fact that these stories reinforce and overlap to a large degree, despite rarely being shared with others, furthers their veracity. Whether in fact every detail is correct, they all fit together surprisingly well. It is essential to remember that God is bigger than we can ever understand.

Notice how commonly Jesus is mentioned in these stories. It is my belief that Jesus far transcends the box that we call "Christianity." Jesus connects in with all religions, and as The Aquarian Gospel elucidates, Jesus can appear to us in any form. In those not familiar with him, as with the little child in the refrigerator, he may appear as a Leprechaun. In someone of another religion, he may appear in a manner that fits in with their spiritual understanding. But, without question, time after time, Jesus is a central theme.

What this book teaches me is that God is incredibly creative, that God has a personality, and that the way insights are shared is in a manner that arouses our curiosity, inspires our witness and increases our yearning to achieve ultimate oneness. Those who persistently seek will find an ever-greater understanding of the incredibly large magnificent puzzle that is God. God wants it to be a giant puzzle. God wants us to use our talents, our skills and our love to solve this ultimate mystery. But what we do know for sure – God is love, we are to love, we are to learn complete forgiveness, we are to be joyful, and that while we are called upon to do great things, it is often the little things that we do every day that make the biggest difference.

<u>My morning affirmations</u> (from Deepak Chopra, Donnie Yance and the Bible)

Every day, in every way, I am increasing my physical, mental and spiritual capacity

Spirituality is the pursuit of holiness

Wipe away the cobwebs of fear, selfishness, greed and narrow-heartedness

This is the most beautiful place in the whole world, right here in Midway, Kentucky!

The more I own, the more it owns me

Am I trusting in God?

Am I allowing my spirit to shine through?

Am I reflecting God, which is love?

This is the day the Lord hath made – rejoice and be glad in it!

"You are my Beloved children. You are named and claimed as my own. You are loved more than you could ever imagine."

-My minister Heather McColl's message from God, 1/11/15, Midway Christian Church, KY

"Religion, in truth, is not a matter of dogmas, beliefs, of rituals and/or superstitions; nor is it the cultivation of personal salvation, for this is a self-centered activity, and a person of religious character is seeking selflessness. Religion is the total way of life for the pursuit of pure Love (God); the inner and outer awareness of the relationship and unity with God, as the Trinity, inclusive of the Cosmos, Nature and Humankind. From within that awareness follows an understanding of the 'Truth' and those challenges, which call us to respond to that Truth, where ALL that we do and are is exemplified as Religion."

-Donnie Yance

Resources

1) **Sign up for Dr. Roach's Health Letter and get two free reports!** 1) Five Natural Ways to Allergy Relief 2) Is 90 percent of Pediatric Medicine Unnecessary? www.themidwaycenter.com

2) **We will offer a free opportunity for you to see or hear interviews** of those you have read about in this book at www.themidwaycenter.com

3) **Is Dr. Roach available to speak?** Yes. Those who pre-purchase books for attendees will be given priority.

4) **Sign up for Don McNay's free reports & Huffington Post articles at** www.huffingtonpost.com/don-mcnay

5) **Can my business benefit from Dr. Roach's knowledge?** Dr. Roach not only educates on the reality of spirituality to optimize focus and cooperation, but also introduces integrative strategies for a full wellness package.

6) **Check for upcoming seminars, webinars, retreats, audio and videos** at www.themidwaycenter.com

7) **Extraordinary Practice Conference** – Nov. 20-21, 2015 for practitioners to optimize knowledge & income www.drroach.net

8) **If I've had these experiences, who can I share them with?** Share these with others who are spiritual; identify them from their sincere, serene, upbeat manner and the positive energy accomplishments in their life. Do not share them with those you perceive as judgmental or negative energy. If you have harmful, fearful or negative energy thoughts, see a spiritual counselor, a minister or integrative health practitioner

9) **Is there a national organization for NDEs?** The International Association of Near-Death Studies www.iands.org

10) **Who are health practitioners I can trust?** The Academy for Integrative Health and Medicine www.aihm.org

11) **What directions should I take for healthcare?** Check the directory of www.aihm.org

12) **What are recommended books?** *Proof of Heaven* by Eban Alexander, M.D., *The Shack* by William P. Young, *Dying to Be Me* by Anita Moorjani

13) **What are tentative topics of Dr. Roach's upcoming books?** The Genius Gene, The Extraordinary Mind, The Extraordinary Pregnancy, Reversing ALS

14) **Would you like to visit Dr. Roach's resort-like hometown?** The Midway website www.meetmeinmidway.com

15) **Would you like to meet spiritualists in the book?** An event can be organized with their presentations

16) For the **Midway Near-Death Experience & Spirituality Support Group:** mhpurdy@gmail.com

17) **How do I attract spiritual experiences into my life?** Through positivity, prayer, faith, humility, compassion, forgiveness, focusing on your positive energy mission, joy, praise, deep gratitude, anonymous generosity and love

18) **Gifted Healers –**
    a. **Michele Waldman:** mwalden444@gmail.com
    b. **Amy Wadel:** www.energybalancehealing.com amydw1@gmail.com
    c. **Beth Bauer:** www.FieldsofEnergy.net
    d. **Dr. Sue Massie, N.D.:** 107 Church Street, Fair Haven, NJ 07704, (732) 933-4011 suemassie45@aol.com
    e. **Ginny Drake:** revisions111@roadrunner.com
    f. **Claudeen Oakley:** itsalifestyleoakley@gmail.com
    g. **Koleoso and Osunnike:** www.manypaths1truth.org 859-225-7769
    h. **Edgar Cayce:** 215 67th Street, Virginia Beach, VA 23451, http://edgarcayce.org/ 800-333-4499

19) **My websites –** www.themidwaycenter.com www.drroach.net

20) **GROW, NURTURE, & CULTIVATE YOUR GIFTS!**

Acknowledgments

My patients' guidance to a "knowing" about God & Jesus
So many beautiful people that I have met in this process
My exceptional office staff, particularly loyal Amy Cress!
Steve Harrison & the Quantum Leap team
Koleoso, Bruce, Marilyn, Lynn, Sue & all contributors!
Kelly Thompson for sage book advice
Office professionals – DeeDee Carman, Wendy Enneking, Lisa
Carson, Angela Rutledge & Lori Rivera
Publishers Don McNay & Adam Turner – outstanding!
Rev. Heather McColl & the Midway Christian Church
My mentors Donnie Yance, Dwight McKee, Bob Anderson & the
whole Mederi/Natura team
Elizabeth & James Roach for writing & tech support
My supportive sister Helen Rentch
My Reiki master Donna Gaines & guide Cyndy Tercha
Hunter Purdy & Deborah for leading the NDE group
My readers including Michelle, Lee, Angela, Sunny & cousin
Margaret Hunter
Rosemary, Beth, Claudean & other spiritual guides
My best friend, John Johnson
Medical partners – Ben Roach, Jack Fisher, Kim Clawson
AIHM with Nan Sudak & Wendy Warner
Spectracell Labs for a chance to prove myself nationally
James Marcum, M.D., Heartwise Ministries for national TV
Andrew Weil, for his nutritional & botanical conferences
My lifetime spiritual guides – Ruth Roach, Searcy Slack, Millard
Fuller, Gandhi, Wayne Dyer & Deepak Chopra

About the Author

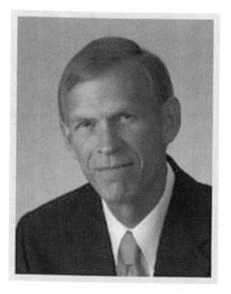

James P. Roach, M.D. (Jim)

Midway Center for Integrative Medicine
www.themidwaycenter.com
www.drroach.net
129 South Winter Street, PO Box 277
Midway, KY 40347-0307
859-846-4445 (work)
859-846-4697 (home)
859-846-4761 (fax)
jproach@aol.com

Midway Family Practice July 1981-2005; renamed:
Midway Center for Integrative Medicine in 2005 – present
Associate Professor, Department of Family and Community
Medicine
University of Kentucky College of Medicine

EDUCATION - BOARD CERTIFICATION
American Board Family Practice Certification
1981
Recertification
1987, 1994, 2001, 2008-15

American Board of Holistic Medicine Certification
2005
Recertification
2012

Tallahassee Memorial Regional Medical Center
Family Practice Residency
1978–81

University of Kentucky College of Medicine
Doctor of Medicine degree
1974–78

Duke University, Durham
Bachelor of Arts degree majoring in Zoology
1970–74

HEALTHCARE PUBLIC SPEAKING
University of KY College of Medicine Family Practice Review:
Tobacco Addiction & Environmental Tobacco Smoke
1998-99

Teaching Patients to Communicate
1999-2000

Teaching Patients to Communicate, Cope & Flourish
2000-2001

Preventive & Complementary Medicine (workshop)
2003-2004

Integrative Solutions in Breast & Prostate Cancer
2007-2008

International Holistic Health Conference
Lexington, KY
Integrative Solutions in Prostate Cancer
2008

2010
1) Annie Appleseed Cancer Project
West Palm Beach, FL
ETMS Approach to Cancer

2) Midway Foundation First Annual Cancer Conference
Lexington, KY
ETMS Approach to Cancer

3) Midway Foundation Fall Conference
Lexington, KY
Integrative Approaches to Degenerative Brain Disorders

2011
1) Midway Foundation's Second Annual Cancer Conference
Lexington, KY
What Experts are Saying

2) Midway Foundation's Fall Conference
Midway College, Midway, KY
Chronic Fatigue and Fibromyalgia

3) Midway Foundation's "Healing Young Brains"
Lexington, KY
Integrative Assessment and Healing of Young Brain Disorders

2012
Advances in Cancer Strategies Symposium
Stamford, CT
ETMS: A Physician's Perspective

2014

Philadelphia, Boston, Chicago, Indianapolis, Columbus OH, Cincinnati, Louisville

Mayo Clinic

National Webinar for Spectracell – record number of listeners

AWARDS

The 1997 Leader in Health Care (in central KY)

The Lane Report

Citations from the Kentucky House, Senate & Governor

2000

PUBLICATIONS

1) Nutrition and Cancer: An International Journal

Volume 65, Issue 5, 2013 pages 653-658

"Differences in Vitamin D Nutritional Status Between Newly Diagnosed Cancer Patients from Rural or Urban Settings in Kentucky"

2) Cancer Strategies Journal

Volume 2, Issue 3, 2014 pages 9-11

"Achieving Peacefulness at Cancer Diagnosis: the Most Important Intervention? – Rationale and Strategies"

PUBLICITY

National Publicity Summit, New York City 2013

National TV: Heartwise Ministries 1hr Call-in 2013

National Radio: KABC Los Angeles 1hr interview 2013

National Speaking: for Spectracell in Philadelphia, Chicago, Boston, Columbus OH, Louisville, Cincinnati 2013-14

Quantum Leap, Philadelphia 2013-15

CONSULTANCY

Spectracell Labs National Consultant 2013-15

BOOKS

Currently planning as of 2015:

THE GENIUS GENE

THE EXTRAORDINARY MIND
THE EXTRAORDINARY PREGNANCY

VOLUNTEER ACTIVITIES
1980-2000
Woodford Habitat for Humanity
Founder 1983
President 1983-88

Chief of Staff, Woodford Hospital
1988 – 1989

Volunteer Faculty Member, Univ. of KY College of Medicine1981-
2014

Kentucky ACTION
(Statewide tobacco control coalition with AHA, ALA, ACS)
Vice Chairperson
1994 – 1996
Chairperson
1996 – 1998

Public speaking:
Radio - Kentucky: WVLK, WHAS
National Radio: Indiana, Pennsylvania, two Internet Stations, KABC
Los Angeles
TV - Kentucky: KET, WAVE, WKYT, WLEX, FOX
National TV – Heartwise Ministries syndicated to 47 states – live
Guest editorials (*Louisville Courier Journal, Lexington Herald
Leader*)

VOLUNTEER ACTIVITIES
2000-2012
President, Woodford Health Alliance
2000-01
Board member, Woodford Health Care
2000-2005
Board member, Woodford Health Foundation

2005-07
Author of the extensive health letter The Transcendent
2004-2007
Scientific Advisory Board for the Mederi Foundation
2007-present
Trustee, Midway College
2001-2015
Midway Foundation for Integrative Medicine
Founder, President 2007-present
UK Markey Cancer Center:
Instigator, Researcher - Study on Cancer Blood Nutritional Markers
Published 2013
Kentucky Lung Cancer Research Board
2009-present
Chairperson 2013-15
American Board of Integrative Holistic Medicine
National test committee
2010-13

NATIONAL CONFERENCES
American Academy of Anti-Aging Medicine conferences
2004, 2005, 2006
Nutrition & Health Conference with Dr. Andrew Weil
University of Arizona
2004, 2005
American Board of Holistic Medicine Conference
2005, 2009, 2010, 2011, 2012, 2013
Botanical Conference, Columbia University
2004
Medicines from the Earth Conferences
2006, 2007, 2009
Amer College for Advancement of Medicine Conf.: Brain Health
2006
Clinical Phytotherapy (Yance)
2006
Family Medicine Board Review
5/2008
Holistic Oncology: The ETMS Approach (Yance)

2007, 2009
Complementary, Preventive, Disease Reversal, & Staying Young
Conference (Cleveland Clinic)
2008
Annie Appleseed Cancer Conference
2010
Midway Foundation Cancer Conference
2010, 2011
Functional Medicine Cancer Symposium
5/2010
Midway Foundation Fall Conference
2010, 10/2011, 2012
Cancer Strategies Conference – Scottsdale, AZ
3/2011
Healing Young Brains – Lexington, KY
11/2011
Advances in Cancer Strategies Symposium
4/2012, 4/2013, 11/2015
American Academy of Environmental Medicine Conference
10/2013
American Holistic Medical Association Conference
10/2014
Extraordinary Practice Conference – organizer & chief presenter
5/2014, 11/2014

Made in the USA
Lexington, KY
09 April 2015